LIVING THE GOOD LIFE

LIVING THE GOOD LIFE

Your Guide to Health and Success

David Patchell-Evans

Foreword by Bill Pearl

ECW PRESS

A percentage of book sales in each country will be donated to help
parents and children with Autism or for Autism research.

This edition published in 2005 by
ECW Press, 2120 Queen Street East, Suite 200, Toronto, Ontario M4E 1E2

ISBN 1-55022-617-7

Patchell-Evans, David
Living the good life : your guide to health and success / David
Patchell-Evans ; foreword by Bill Pearl.

1. Physical fitness. 2. Health. 3. Success. 4. Patchell-Evans, David. I. Title.

RA776.P374 2003   613.7   C2003-903127-6

10 9 8 7 6

JACKET DESIGN: BILL DOUGLAS @ THE BANG
TEXT DESIGN AND PAGE COMPOSITION: PAGEWAVE GRAPHICS INC.

PRINTED AND BOUND IN CANADA

ECW PRESS
ecwpress.com

To my mom, Dorothy, for everything,
who after 80 years and death-defying surgery
finally got a personal trainer.

To Jane, my indispensable second-in-charge
for 20 years and who I consider to be a sister
by rites of passage.

To my brothers Ed and Jerry for always being there.

To Kilamanjaro and Tygre-Joy,
my two precious daughters, who enlighten
and enrich my life beyond measure.

Contents

FOREWORD

I FIRST MET David Patchell-Evans almost two decades ago, when
he became a customer of the company I work for, which
specializes in electronic fitness equipment and for which
I'm a national spokesperson in the United States. Since
that time I've had the pleasure of attending conferences
with "Patch" and I've been a keynote speaker at several
GoodLife Fitness Clubs educational events.

Even though I have spent many hours with him, I
really didn't get to know the true Patch until I had the
pleasure of reading this book, *Living the Good Life*. It
was an eye-opener. In real life Patch is a very private person, the opposite of me. I am a much better talker than I
am a listener, so I had never heard his full story until sitting down with this book.

I have followed Patch's career in the fitness industry and have watched the amazing growth of his business, but I could never put my finger on exactly what it
was that made him so successful. This book gives the
answer — Dave Patchell-Evans loves people more than
he loves money.

I should have known this long before reading his book, because I have been on the receiving end of his kindness many times over the years. One example of this was his buying hundreds of copies of my various fitness books to give away as gifts. Another is that I have never attended any function of his where he has not tried to give me the centre spotlight.

I have been in the health-club business for over 50 years. I have run gyms in California for over 30 years, and have personally coached more major contest-winners than almost anyone else in fitness history: ten Mr. Universe titles, eight Mr. America titles, and one Mr. Olympia title. When I met Patch I knew that he was someone very special indeed. Believe me, people like Patch are unique in the fitness industry. He has compassion for all his club members, and his goal is to make every one of them a success story — on their own terms.

An example of how he goes about this comes from personal observation. I have seen Patch call person after person by their first names as he walks through his clubs. And I have seen the payback, when members do the same to him (I have never heard anyone call him Mr. Patchell-Evans). People feel good in his presence. They come to believe they can be fit and healthy, even if they've never exercised a day in their lives until then.

Patch is great at convincing people that it's fun and easy to become fit.

One of the many things Patch has done by writing this book is to show anyone who is able to move that there is hope for a better day. He has put his thoughts in lay language. And the best part is that he tells you the truth. You do not have to spend hours a day doing something you don't like in order to make progress.

Patch writes from the heart. I believe him when he says his goal is to make every person he comes into contact with feel better about life. Wouldn't it be nice if the whole world were filled with people like Dave Patchell-Evans? I know one thing — as a population we would all be a lot happier and healthier if he had his way.

It is my hope that you will be touched by the warmth and encouragement of Patch's words, and that you'll realize that you too can live the good life.

BILL PEARL
FIVE-TIME MR. UNIVERSE WINNER

PREFACE

I WROTE THIS book because I want to encourage you to live the good life. What is the good life? It's about health. It's about feeling at home in your body. It's about allowing your body to become the best it can be. It's the feeling of energy and alertness you feel when you're in good shape. It's about the confidence with which you meet life challenges. It's knowing that you can achieve far more than you ever dreamed of. It's the sense of yourself as a body, mind, heart, and soul — a whole being, vibrant and alive.

Contrary to what we're told by media and even fitness "gurus," being healthy and fit is not difficult. It's easy. I hope I can convince you in these pages just how easy it is. And when you experience how easy it is, you'll also experience how joyful and life-affirming it is to feel your health improve and the mastery of your life increase.

Writing this book has been a journey — a journey of putting down onto paper the thoughts and feelings I have carried about fitness for a long time, the thoughts and feelings that drive the success of GoodLife Fitness Clubs and my own personal life. I could not have made this journey into the demanding world of book publishing without the help and support of many individuals.

My thanks to:

Sharon Lindenburger, who functioned as my trusted "scribe." Sharon, a health-care journalist and author in her own right, helped me distill the wisdom of my thoughts and express them in a way that is accessible to readers from all walks of life. Her expertise in writing is reflected in the pages of this book.

Megan Cameron, GoodLife's Director of Communications, who kept the project on track, kept me motivated to get this book done, and encouraged me while she took care of all the myriad details of gathering information and facilitating meetings among key people.

Don Bastian, of Bastian Publishing Services, who believed in this project and who guided the creation of the book with great care, sensitivity, and patience.

Bill Pearl, who has been an inspiration to me from the beginnings of my career in the fitness industry, and who kindly agreed to write the foreword to this book.

Barry "Bears" Neil Kaufman, for the insights that our company and I use from his book *Happiness Is a Choice*.

And all the wonderful GoodLife staff, its consultants, and the following upper management: Jane Riddell, Dorothy Walsh, Maureen Hagan, Sue Chambers, Wes Shaver, Kathy Kaye, Ryan DiPede, Michele Colwell,

Eric Slota, Marian McTeer, Shelley Ramsay, Collette Watts, Dawn Underwood, Bill and Toni Van Haeren, Mike Chaet, Deb Smith, Judi Ohm, Phil Sorrell, Brian Mortimer, Peter Rasimus, Sharilyn Aitken, Ian Blair, Megan Cameron, Brad Lindsay, Sue Marsh, Andy Thompson, Lindy Brecht, and Dann Sawa, whose dedication to delivering our programs and caring for our members make GoodLife one of the top fitness club chains in North America, indeed in the world.

I would also like to recognize the long-time dedication of my professional advisers, Henry Berg, Bill Shanks, and Jay Trothen.

And finally, I'd like to thank GoodLife's members, especially those who openly share their personal stories in this book. These stories touched my heart, as they affirm so many of the positive things that can happen in people's lives when they take control of their health and fitness. Without our thousands of wonderful members, GoodLife would not exist. And so, to you, the members of GoodLife, 100,000 strong and growing, I say: YOU are the reason I wrote this book. I could not have done it without you.

"Patch"
DAVID PATCHELL-EVANS

LIVING THE GOOD LIFE

CHAPTER ONE

THE SIMPLICITY OF BEING FIT

WHY IS IT that only one out of five people — 20 percent of the population — exercises regularly? Why do the other 80 percent not bother? Why are they mainly sedentary, or think physical activity is taking out the garbage every Wednesday night? It's because they think fitness is hard. They think they can't do it or that they don't have time to do it. But I'm here to tell you that it's easy, and that you can do it. The whole point of this book is to make you realize how simple it is to be fit — and what you will gain in your life from becoming fit and healthy.

I'm not a "fitness guru." I'm not going to tell you about the latest fad diets or give you detailed descriptions of complicated exercises and fitness equipment. I'm going to tell you some of what I've learned in my more than 20 years in the fitness industry. I'm a person who cares very much about well-being and health. I want to see a society in which greater numbers of people achieve total well-being. I want to see people make decisions for health and vitality. I want to play a part in helping them put those decisions into action. This is the driving vision of my entire professional life.

It's this passion for health and fitness — and the knowledge that it's simple — that has led my company, GoodLife Fitness Clubs Inc., to become the largest chain of fitness facilities in Canada and one of the largest in North America. We have over 50 clubs, with more coming on board every month, almost 2,000 employees, and over 100,000 members and growing. And we have only one reason for being — to make you fit and healthy, to make you believe you can do this, to get you off the couch and into your own body.

My Own Journey into Fitness

MY OWN LEVEL of activity as a child was not all that unusual. I didn't spend my childhood as an athlete in training. In the High Park area of Toronto where I grew up, I was just a regular active kid. I played hockey, went to summer camps, and spent time at the family cottage up until about age 12, when I became old enough to begin summer jobs. I always had jobs that required physical labour. I rode a bicycle to make deliveries for a drugstore. I worked at a gas station — I used to make a game of how fast I could run from one car to another to pump the gas, jumping between the gas pumps and swinging on them. What I didn't realize about the bicycling and the gas station antics was that what I was doing was aerobic "training." The High Park area is really hilly, and biking up and down those slopes every night from 4 p.m. to 8 p.m. got my legs into great shape.

A little later, when I became interested in rowing and was trying out for the national team, my bicycling experience served me well. The team recruiters used to test prospective rowers on a bicycle, and I was one of the best. It was that summer job doing drugstore deliveries that helped open the door for me to become a Canadian team champion rower later on.

You might think that doing such physical jobs would put the idea of "fitness" in my head, but it didn't. It wasn't until I was in a physical rehab clinic, totally torn apart, that I began to understand what the body needs to be healthy. At age 19, during my second week of university, I had a serious motorcycle accident. A car cut me off and the motorcycle I was riding fell on top of me. In one of those bursts of strength you get when you're in an emergency and your nerves are all fired up, I threw the motorcycle off me. I couldn't move for several hours after that. My clavicle was broken. My shoulder was dislocated, tendons and muscles torn. I was a total mess. I ended up going for rehabilitation at the renowned Fowler-Kennedy clinic at the University of Western Ontario in London, Ontario, where I was a student. (Dr. Pete Fowler now has a clinic in one of my clubs — it's a relationship that goes back 25 years.)

While I was at the clinic, I watched people in all stages of rehabilitation, some recovering from accidents far more severe than mine had been. For the first time I became aware of the fragility of life, how limited and finite it is — and not just life, but quality of life. To me these two things are similar, but also very different. One is about staying alive. If you've had a stroke or a heart attack, or if you've been in a car accident, you're happy just to be alive. You say to yourself, "Thank God, I'm still here." But then you get to rehab and the question becomes, "What's the quality of my life going to be?"

There I was, almost 20, and I had to ask myself, "Am I going to have one shoulder four inches lower than the other, or am I going to get into shape and build it back up?" In the clinic I was surrounded by people all going through the trauma of some kind of injury. At the same time, the top athletes at UWO would come to the clinic to use the equipment because it was so much more advanced than anything else available at the time. So, right beside me, really motivated athletes would be working out. There were also athletes who had been injured, and they were the most motivated of all. I took all this in and thought about it at length. As a young university student I was also at the stage of pondering, "What am I going to do with my life? What career do I want?" At the clinic I saw the satisfaction that arises from looking after others, helping make sure they have a decent quality of life, even in the face of accidents and injuries.

For the rest of that school year, I did rehab and tried to get back into shape. That summer I first got a job as a lumberjack and then later as a lifeguard. In the fall I took up rowing. I had come to UWO to go to its business school. I also took a physical education course, but at first I didn't take it all that seriously. But it turned out to be very interesting, and in second year I took another physical education course. That course was instrumental in forming my ideas about the direction I wanted to go. The course instructors kept touching on the benefits to your head and your heart that come from doing physical activity. I ended up switching from the business school into physical education.

During that third year I rowed competitively, and took another course on the philosophy of physical education, given by Jack Fairs. Jack kept talking about how, through most of history, people have thought of the body as one thing, the mind as another, and the soul as still another. His point was that they're really the same thing, and he would give example after example. I thought he was a great instructor, despite the fact that I sometimes fell asleep in his class because I had been out snowplowing the night before. That was another hat I wore in university: I started a snowplowing business and it paid my way through school. It provided much needed cash and, most important, a credit rating.

I also took business planning courses at UWO's business school. One course was an exploration of what kind of business I would like to establish. I did my business plan on how to open a squash club. I had come to realize that I wanted to do something in the recreation/ fitness field. I wanted to make a difference for people, using my skills — to be the initiator of a fitness-related business and create opportunities for people to lead healthy lives. What you learn in business school doesn't often prepare you to be your own boss. You learn skills that enable you to work for someone else who has a vision. The people who own companies are the ones with vision. They hire people with business degrees to help run their companies. I wanted both the vision and the ability to run my own company.

It occurred to me that there was nobody out there with a vision about fitness who knew anything about business. So I decided to put the two together — I had the physical education training and the business training, and then I worked hard at developing salesmanship. I took courses such as exercise physiology, scientific training techniques, dance, racquetball, and so forth — things that would enable me to run a club. I knew how to make the body go fast and I understood a balance sheet. In the meantime, I had continued rowing, and ended up winning five Canadian championships. Then I tried out for the 1980 Olympics. The year before the Games, the national team suggested to the Olympic candidates that we work out on Nautilus equipment. Up to then I had been lifting free weights, but when I was in rehab I had used Nautilus equipment for my injured shoulders, so off I went to a fitness club that had the equipment. Every day while I was working out I would ask the owner questions about his business. One day he said to me, "If you're so interested in this club, why don't you buy it? It's for sale."

I said, "No problem. I'll come back at nine o'clock and we'll talk about it." I came back at nine with a 12-pack of beer, by midnight we had made a deal, and the next morning when the club opened, I was the owner.

By then I had completed a year of my master's degree, but I had taken a year off to train for the Olympics. Actually, the university told me to take the year off because they felt my priorities weren't straight. I ran a snowplowing business, which had grown considerably. I had five trucks, about a dozen employees, and 120 lots to plow every time it snowed — I made good money. I was also a carded athlete, receiving some government funding for my training, and I had a paying teaching assistantship as part of my master's program.

In December of 1977 it snowed like crazy. I snowplowed every single night for three weeks and slept only every second day for three or four hours. I made a lot of money, but I feel asleep during two of my exams. The professors thought that I had my priorities all wrong, that I was more focused on making money than on my studies. In March they told me to take the year off to think. I took the summer off, rowed in the fall, and got my snow-plowing business organized for another winter. I took lots of holidays and I trained.

In April of the following year came the opportunity to buy the club. The money I had made the previous year gave me enough capital. The club was called Canada Pro Fitness at Adelaide and Cheapside Streets in London, Ontario. That was my first club, the forerunner of the GoodLife Fitness Clubs chain.

In doing the business plan for that first club, I discovered that no one in fitness clubs knew anything about fitness! Their focus was on sales. They were business people. And at the universities, where all the physical education specialists were, no one knew anything about sales. The opportunity presented to me was to become someone who could learn about sales, who could know about business and about fitness, and who had a passion for making people better. I had reached a high level of fitness through my rowing and my physical education courses, and had experienced physical recovery in rehab. I had a good idea of what was necessary to achieve a high quality of life in terms of exercise and fitness.

It Makes Perfect Sense

YOU DECIDE HOW fit you're going to be. This was the core philosophy of GoodLife right from that very first club: to give you the control and the means to achieve a healthy body and a sharp mind. You can make a conscious decision about how well you want to be, and that decision will affect your whole quality of life. Six months after my injury I was working as a lumberjack, then as a lifeguard. Ten months later I was part of a competitive rowing team. Those were my choices. Not everyone has to pursue a sport. That was just my particular spin on things. We're going to talk a lot more about the differences between athletics and fitness later on in this book.

It was only a few years ago that medical associations in the United States and Canada began saying that fitness actually increases the length of your life. From my own experience I knew that fitness made people better. I knew it made them happier. I knew it gave them more energy, made them more optimistic, and improved their self-esteem. It just made sense that fitness would also help people live longer. We all know that if we treat a car well and keep it well maintained, it will last longer. But we don't seem to understand that about our own bodies. We've known for hundreds of years that how well you treat a horse determines how well the horse rides. If you had a horse worth $100,000 you'd give it the best food, you would make sure it got good exercise, you would look after its health. Most people don't do that for themselves. Most people don't think they're worth as much as a $100,000 horse.

When I opened my first fitness club, it made sense to me to take advantage of this opportunity. Although fitness clubs had existed for a while, they were called "health spas," and the emphasis was on passivity and relaxation. There's nothing wrong with relaxation, but the other side of the equation is activity. You don't get to relax and enjoy your paycheque until you've worked. With fitness, you have to put in a little effort before you get to the "relax and enjoy" part. But the really neat thing about fitness is that you don't have to spend a lot of time to get unbelievable benefits. You do have to continue with it — it can't be just a "sometime" thing. We have to eat all the time; we have to bathe all the time. Fitness doesn't take any more time than preparing a meal or taking a bath. If you spend half an hour three times a week doing fitness activities, you'll be in better shape than 90 percent of the population.

Another advantage I had from my training background was that I realized there are other options than just lifting barbells. There is more than one way to shape up your heart and lungs. There is more than one way to build up your muscles. And now science and technology have made it even easier, because we've got exercise equipment today that didn't exist even five years ago. If you can get to the point where you are exercising three times a week for six months — whether by using equipment or by other means — you will know and understand the benefits of fitness, because you'll feel these benefits. You'll feel them in your body and you'll feel them in your spirit. And you'll keep on doing it.

Turning Point

I DON'T WANT to imply that if you take the road to fitness you will never have any rough times. Life can hit us broadside with things we don't expect. It's a matter of deciding that, no matter what happens, you will be the best you can be. The accident I had when I was 19 was a turning point in my life, because if I hadn't gone through rehab and been turned on to fitness I would just have gone into the business world. But another, even more dramatic turning point happened when I was 32.

I had been competing in the World Masters' Rowing Championships and had won three medals. When I woke up the next morning, I couldn't get out of bed. I couldn't carry my gym bag, I couldn't open the door, I couldn't turn the key in the car ignition. I had to walk on the sides of my feet because they were so painful. I couldn't put my elbows on the table because they had grown by two inches, full of lumpy mush. I had bumps all over my body. At work someone had to help me lift the lightest weight. I couldn't turn the bicycle wheels. I owned about seven or eight clubs at the time, all of which demanded my attention, and I felt as if I was falling apart. I was in tremendous pain.

No one could diagnose the problem at first. I tried massage and chiropractic, but nothing helped. About two months after this nightmare began, my mother became ill and I took her to the hospital. The doctor on call was Duncan McKinley, who had been a friend of mine at university and had played in the Canadian Football League. We needed to adjust my mother's position on the bed to make her more comfortable. Duncan asked me to help, but I fumbled, unable to lift my mother. He asked, "What's wrong?"

I said, "I can't use my hands."

He looked at my hands and then back at me, and replied, "Well, Patch, you've got arthritis."

No one had picked up on this, because you don't expect "Mr. Fitness Guy" to have arthritis. Duncan sent me to some specialists for tests, and they found the RA factor in my blood — I had rheumatoid arthritis.

The first thing they told me was not to exercise. I paid attention to that advice for about a month, but the only thing that happened was that I got weaker. I had weighed about 210 pounds on a six-foot-five frame and was pretty strong, and my weight dropped to 180 pounds just from muscle wasting away. So I disobeyed doctors' orders and started to exercise. At first I had to get someone to help me just move at all — a form of personal training in its infancy. Gradually I got to the point where I could turn the bicycle wheel by myself and work through the pain. And when I did that, I felt better afterwards.

The doctors tried different drugs on me. I learned all about arthritis attacks, how they come in cycles. I experimented with nutrition and worked my way right through the medical library looking up information on rheumatoid arthritis. What I found was that mental attitude makes a huge difference. The same skills that you need as a business person to be successful, and that you need as an athlete to excel, you must apply to healing your body. My illness, and my efforts to cope with it and break through it, taught me the most important lesson about fitness and about running a fitness-oriented business.

That big door that opened for me was a far greater understanding about not taking things for granted. When I was having constant pain with every motion, I no longer took movement for granted. This pushed me to a whole new level in terms of my humanity and empathy. Now I understand when a 79-year-old person comes into one of my clubs and says, "I can't do stuff." Or someone comes in after having surgery and says, "I'm having trouble recuperating." Or a person says, "I've weighed 40 pounds too much for a long time and I just can't seem to lose it." I have an idea of how hard it is. Very few people in the fitness industry really understand what it's like to be old or weakened. But I became "old" at 32, and I had to work to recover the quality of life I valued. This has made an enormous difference in how I run my clubs and how I have designed my business to take care of people's needs.

"Be the Best You Can Be"

THE EMPHASIS IN fitness, as I see it, is to train people for success, their success. The purpose is not to make judgements, but to help each person become the best he or she can be. I know this is a cliché we hear bandied about by motivational speakers and in self-help books — "Be the best you can be" — but the fact that it's an overworked phrase doesn't make it less true. To me, being the best you can be means becoming as highly functioning as possible, and not just physically. Exercise makes you smarter — you're getting more oxygen to the brain. There are studies showing that children who exercise at school get better marks. It's not a big jump to say that working people who exercise get better money. Studies show that physically active people are more productive and have far fewer absences from work. If you know that fitness makes you feel better — makes you be better — then it can encourage you not to accept mediocrity in yourself, and that will have positive effects in many areas of your life. But you will only reach the "better" when you push the basics. You will only know what it's like to be good at something, to achieve your own personal best — not compared to anyone else — if you push your own limits. And your limits are just things you're used to.

A couple of years ago I went climbing by myself in Palm Springs. I had noticed some small mountains nearby. I hadn't done any real climbing since I got arthritis, but they didn't look that high. I left the hotel at 5:30 a.m. and began the climb. It was really steep, and before long I was clambering over rocks and boulders, wondering what on earth I was trying to prove — it was like being on nature's StairMaster. The sun was rising behind me when all of a sudden I saw a glint higher up. A coyote was looking down at me from 75 feet above. The sunlight had caught its fur and made it shine golden. It was the most beautiful sight, and I would never have seen it if I hadn't pushed myself to try that climb. On my way back down there were more coyotes, watching me from a distance.

I was back for breakfast at 9 a.m. Do you think the other hotel guests had any clue what I had just enjoyed? It couldn't have happened if I hadn't had a good fitness level, developed through exercising six times a week, half an hour a day, for the previous 10 years. It doesn't even have to be six times a week. You can exercise three times a week and still be amazingly fit. Two days after I saw the coyotes, I climbed up by the gondola in Palm Springs and did my very first overhang — scary, challenging, and rewarding. I can still remember that feeling of accomplishment.

It's all about gaining a sense of control over yourself. I won't say control over your life, because many things happen to us in life that we can't control. But you can have control of yourself and how you respond to those things. When people first come into a fitness club, many have never done exercise. They've never participated in any kind of physical activity. Fitness gives you control. Your body will degenerate if you don't use it, but if you exercise you don't have to get old. Everyone ages, but if you're fit you're going to age a lot more slowly.

A lot of self-help methods are based on mental discipline, or on working through emotional issues so that you see them in a new light, or on doing spiritual work such as learning forgiveness and compassion. But what these approaches lack is that they don't get the body into the equation. The health of your body influences what you experience in your mind. There is no split. If you can engage your whole spirit in the pursuit of fitness — not just your intellect, not just your emotions — you'll discover what it is to be a whole person.

Your body needs and wants exercise. It needs it every 48 hours just to recover from the stresses of everyday life. It needs it to maintain strong bones. It needs it to have a lower heart rate. It needs it so that you don't have fatty acids in your arteries. Your head needs it: If you burn off stress, you think more clearly. All these things allow your soul to be free, because you feel "in sync."

Best Doesn't Mean Perfect

ONE THING THAT I think is really important in the field of fitness is that it's not about perfection. Being your best, in terms of fitness, is not about being perfect. We all know of people who go overboard, who seem totally addicted to exercise and do it for hours every day. But such obsessive exercisers are few in the overall population. There are a lot fewer compulsive exercisers than there are compulsive overeaters. There are a lot fewer compulsive exercisers than there are compulsive workers, compulsive worriers, or compulsive TV watchers.

At GoodLife I have a saying: "Enough is enough." What we try to do is help establish a person's objectives. You might say, for example, "I want to lose 10 pounds, have a resting heart rate of 60 beats per minute, and be able to play with my kids without getting tired out." You establish these things as goals and make a time frame in which to get them done.

When you've reached your goals, you have three choices. First, you can pat yourself on the back, go home, and do nothing further, which means that in the same time it took to get you into shape you'll also get out of shape again. A lot of people think fitness is something you achieve and then it just stays there. That's not true.

The second choice is to say "enough is enough" and then maintain the gains. You've reached your goals and you have enough energy. All you have to do is show up three times a week to exercise, and you'll keep your level of fitness. For example, if you do 20 minutes on the stair machine and eight strength exercises that work the whole body, three times a week, that's all you'll have to do forever. That's phenomenally easy.

The hard part is the first six months — but anyone can do six months, when you really think about it. This psychology is foreign to our culture. Most people think, "As soon as I've got to here, I've got to get to *there*." You don't have to. We know that if you do two good strength workouts a week, it will help you get stronger. And if you do three cardiovascular workouts a week, you'll keep your heart and lungs in good shape.

The third choice is the constant struggle to be better, to keep pushing. If I can walk a hundred feet, then I can go a thousand feet, then 10,000 feet. Then I have to run a thousand feet, then 10,000 feet. That's well and good if you want to do that. But you don't have to. All you have to do is work to get your optimum level of fitness for you, and then maintain it. You don't have to keep pushing, unless you want to.

Let's say you get on a fitness machine and you move

20 pounds for two weeks. Then you decide to try 22 pounds. My job as a fitness professional might be to tell you that, for you, 22 is fine. You might think, "I've run three miles. Now I have to run 10." You don't. Anything you run after three miles would be for your own personal satisfaction. It's not because you need it for your fitness. The physiological difference between two hours of running and just half an hour is between 2 and 5 percent. Do you burn more fat? Yes. Does your heart get more efficient? Yes — but only marginally. You don't have to become an exercise fanatic in order to enjoy the phenomenal benefits that fitness will give you.

Another issue that affects your ability to be your best is time. People often say, "I don't have time to exercise." Yet numerous studies have shown that, at a minimum, you are 20 percent more productive if you exercise. If you're 20 percent more productive, that means you create 33 more hours per week by exercising. Where do the 33 hours come from? You get them because your decisions are 20 percent faster, you have 20 percent less anxiety, your sleep is 20 percent deeper. You create time by exercising. If you exercise for half an hour three times a week, you gain the equivalent of 33 hours a week in terms of productivity. You give up an hour and a half to gain 33. By avoiding fitness, you're not saving any time. You're actually losing it. Invariably, people who are leaders in business, politics, sports, and life in general are physically active.

We Are
Physical Beings

FITNESS MAKES YOU centred. Fitness underlines the reality that you are a physical being. It wasn't all that long ago that we were hunters and gatherers and our survival depended on our bodies' ability to move and be flexible and strong. You are built for physical activity. If you don't do it, you can create disease. When you don't participate in activity, you are working counter to your body, which means that you are lowering the quality of every other aspect of your life.

In these times of rapid technological change, which hasn't even begun to peak yet, people often feel out of control, powerless to stop change or to navigate through it. Stress is an epidemic in this society. But the things you definitely can control are your attitude and your body. You decide if you're going to be happy. You decide if you're going to be fit. Get rid of all the absolutes. I don't know of many people who think they have perfect bodies. When I give a staff seminar to 1,400 people and ask which of them has a perfect body, few people are bold enough to stick their hands up. The question has to be "Who is happy with their body?" Still, most people wouldn't put their hands up on that one either, because everyone thinks his or her body has to be better. And people who you think have perfect bodies aren't always happy with their bodies, either. We have to get away from this need for perfection to "it's right for me."

It All Comes Together

THE ACCIDENT I had when I was 19 made me aware that there are "roses," things in life to be savoured. Life had to be more than just survival. There had to be quality of life. But it wasn't until I got sick with rheumatoid arthritis that I really figured out the concept of the "soul" in fitness. It wasn't until every movement hurt that I understood my body's role in nurturing my spirit. The best thing that ever happened to me was getting arthritis. It awakened me to how good every single moment is. It made me realize that caring for my body, giving it the activity it needs — even when the pain is so great I think, "No way am I doing this" — this is the very best thing I can do for myself. Positive adherence to physical activity is food that brings balance to the soul, the intellect, the heart, and the body. It puts it all together. At some deep, basic level we all know this. We know it, but most of us don't do anything about it.

In the rest of this book we're going to talk about how we get from knowing to doing. Knowing that something is good for you is not enough to make you do it. You have to feel good doing it. Along the way we'll share some experiences of people who have gone from knowing to doing, stories of ordinary people, not athletic superstars, who came into GoodLife Fitness Clubs looking for a way to enhance their health and well-being and made amazing gains.

When it comes to fitness, the human body is a pleasure-seeking organism. We'll only do it if it feels good. But it's not the desire to feel good that initially motivates most people to try exercise. It's the desire to look good. So that's where we'll begin in the next chapter — talking about looking good.

CHAPTER TWO

LOOKING GOOD

MOST PEOPLE JOIN a fitness club because they don't like the way they look. They want to look better. In a culture that values physical appearance, it's small wonder that very few of us are happy with the bodies we have. There's nothing wrong with wanting to look good. But in this chapter I want to expand the idea of looking good, so that we can use this very human desire to be attractive and appealing to others to help us arrive at more important and lasting reasons to pursue regular fitness activities.

Looking good requires a balance between your body type and your self-image, whereas a good weight is the most functionally healthy weight for you. These two aspects may not be in sync. For example, one woman might think she looks really good when she is phenomenally thin. If she takes that to an extreme, she becomes anorexic. Most anorexics are women — not all, but most — because the onus on women at this particular time in history has been to be slimmer, slimmer, slimmer. So a woman may look in the mirror and think, "I'm fat," when in fact her body weight may be exactly what it's supposed to be.

On the other side of the scale, a man wants to have bigger, bigger, bigger muscles. He may look in the mirror and see not a hulk with muscles coming out of his earlobes but a skinny guy who is scared to walk down the beach. So, just as a woman may feel that being thin makes people think more highly of her, a man thinks that bigger muscles will make people think more highly of him. A man might be motivated to take drugs to enhance his muscle size. A woman might be motivated to take diuretics to decrease her body size.

All of this happens because we've bought into cultural ideals of "female beauty" and "manliness" that are not based in the reality of who we are — human beings with varying body types.

Your Body Type Determines How You Look

LOOKING GOOD IS about being comfortable in your own skin and realizing that your body type, what scientists call your somatotype, determines much of the way you look. Even if you totally accept your body type and make your body the best for that type, you will never reach "perfection." But you can get 95 percent of what you want with half an hour of exercise three times a week.

There are three main body types: ectomorph, endomorph, and mesomorph. An ectomorph is a linear person. He or she tends to be tall, with long limbs, a slender trunk, a smaller chest frame, hip girdle, and hip bones, and narrow shoulders. An endomorph is a round person. He or she has round thighs, round arms, a round face, and a round chest. A mesomorph has a larger chest, smaller hips, and large shoulders, and seems to be muscular without doing anything. Everyone is a combination of these different types, but most of us tend to be predominantly one type.

When these various body types exercise, the ectomorph gains some muscle and becomes more functionally strong, the endomorph loses some roundness and puts on some muscle, and the mesomorph becomes more dramatically muscular. These different body types excel at different sports. Endomorphs or mesomorphs may be better at swimming because they have more body fat to help support them in the water, but a long, linear ectomorph will flourish as a rower.

Evolution Plays
a Role

YOU CAN'T FIGHT Mother Nature. Genetically, males and females have differing tendencies. Down through history, at least until the Industrial Revolution, females tended to be the gatherers of food. They didn't run as much and they bore children. They carried the loads of food and children, so heavier hips became a physical adaptation over thousands of years. As a result of this evolutionary pattern, women came to carry fat first and foremost on their derrieres and their thighs, where it didn't interfere with gathering or with having children. When a woman didn't have reliable food sources and had to store fat, the derriere and the thighs were the safest places to store it. So the first place a woman puts weight on is where she doesn't want it, because it sticks right out. And when she undertakes to lose weight, the derriere and the thighs will be the last places it seems to come off. If you're a woman and you've got extra weight on your abdomen, it can be lost quite easily, but you'll go crazy waiting for it to come off your derriere.

Now let's look at the men. The average man carries extra weight on his abdomen. Thousands of years ago the men were hunters. They had to be able to run, either toward something or away from something. The best place to store fat and not have it interfere with running is your stomach. Your vital organs are in that area as well, so if something did happen, you had all that fat to protect you. The second place a man puts on weight is his back, where it also acts as protection and doesn't get in the way. If you're doing activities with your upper body, such as hitting, punching, or throwing, and you have too much fat on your arms, you can't function as quickly. This is Nature's way of looking after you if you're a man — by storing the fat on your abdomen and back.

Men have to be careful to avoid being unrealistic about wanting to have a "washboard stomach," where you can see all the abdominal muscles. If the average male gets down to the point of showing his abdominal muscles, it means he has about 6 to 8 percent body fat. Some men would have to go to 4 percent, which is too low. A small number of men can show those muscles at 10 percent body fat. What men need to realize is that they won't get those "perfect abs" until their body fat, as a whole, is low and they've toned up their whole bodies. This is nearly impossible for many men, and some endanger their health by reducing their body fat to too low a level.

Taking all this into account, you still want to achieve the best for yourself in terms of your appearance. The key thing to realize is that you are making yourself look good primarily to please yourself, and only secondarily to please others. We've got it backwards in this society. We seek to impress others, but we're not impressed with ourselves. If you can make yourself happy and comfortable in your own body, in most cases what other people think won't matter. Being the body type you are, accepting your somatoform and working with it, allows you the freedom to enjoy your life.

Two Components of Looking Good

LOOKING GOOD INVOLVES two distinct components. One is feeling good about yourself just for participating in physical activity, feeling good about every improvement you make, as opposed to thinking you will only look good when you're perfect. I remember training for the 1980 Olympics. At that stage I was in the best shape of my life. I weighed 215 pounds, with 8 percent body fat. But I worked out six hours a day, I ate like crazy, and that's all I did. There was no way I could do all the other things I wanted to do. For most of us, that trade-off in the pursuit of a perfect body is just not workable. The key to looking good is being prepared to thank yourself for every improvement you make, to see yourself in the mirror and know that you look as good as you did last year. Given the fact that most people get older, it's a good thing if — through exercise — you can look the same from one year to the next. You're slowing down your aging.

The second aspect of looking good is when people say to you, "You look good." To get this response, you need the strength to have good posture. You need the cardiovascular capacity not to look tired. You need flexibility in your joints so that you don't become old before your time. The act of exercising creates energy, and as you create energy you give your body vitality. And if you have vitality, you look good.

What happens when you get fit is that you become comfortable with yourself. As that comfort level goes up, you will gradually transform yourself into what you want to be, within your own capabilities. You're exercising and all of a sudden your muscles feel firmer, you hold your head a little higher, your posture improves, your joints are aligned, and you carry your weight better — even if it's the same weight you had when you began. Your skin starts to get better. Your respiration improves. Exercise speeds up elimination of toxins from the body.

I like to use plumbing as an analogy. Exercise cleans out your plumbing. Most people understand that clean water in a house comes in through the pipes and dirty water goes out through the sewer. Think of your veins as sewers and your arteries as fresh-water pipes. Oxygen comes into your lungs, your blood picks up the oxygen, and the heart pumps that clean blood through your arteries (the arteries are an excellent transport system). The veins take the blood minus the oxygen back to the lungs to be renewed.

What happens when you exercise is that your arteries and veins expand and contract with greater elasticity.

Exercise burns up some of the waste products created by various bodily functions. As it burns them up, it cleans your arteries and veins and the blood moves more easily. And the lungs, when you exercise, take in oxygen more efficiently. You get more fresh air to your head and body. As a result, you can think better, which is why there is a correlation between exercise and intelligence.

Every Part Is Meant for Exercise

EVERY PART OF your body is meant for exercise. Your body is meant to function, not just to be passive. You start to exercise and your body says, "Hey, I don't feel bad." Say, for example, you're a person who is not that physically active. But one night you go out to a party and you dance maybe a dozen dances. Then you come home and take a nice warm shower. Chemicals called endorphins kick into your bloodstream, and your body says, "I'm making you feel good because I'm hoping you'll do this again tomorrow." While you were dancing, you burned off some of the negative, stress-producing chemicals in your body.

After you break the cycle of inactivity, sometime between six weeks and six months later you will start to feel the pleasure of exercise, and your body will tell you, "This is good." If this is the case, how come that night of dancing doesn't cause you to run right out and join a fitness club or buy some exercise equipment for your home? The reason lies again in our evolutionary patterns. Because, throughout most of human history, people often didn't have enough food, or at least no consistent supply of food, we evolved to store and conserve fat so that when we needed it, we had it. That's not an issue anymore — most of us don't have to worry about starvation. In North America we usually have to worry about the opposite — overeating.

But the body is still in the "conserve energy" mode. If you're just sitting on your couch, your body slips back into the mode of "There might be a hurricane tomorrow and maybe I won't be able to get food, so I'd better save my energy." But the fact of the matter is that, since you do have enough food, the very act of doing something physical creates more energy. That's why exercise makes you feel energetic. It's self-perpetuating. We all think the remedy for stress is to relax. But physical activity will create the energy so that we can relax. It's a paradox: Be active and you will relax more deeply. But if you're a couch potato, all your relaxation will simply make you more tired.

The big challenge in looking good for your body type is realizing that you have to beat your habitual urge to do nothing, so that you become a participant in life instead of a victim waiting for the floods to come. The key issue in looking good is realizing that you will never be totally satisfied with how you look. Don't get caught on the perfection treadmill. You'll drive yourself crazy and you'll quit. And then you'll never break the bad habit of inactivity.

At age 45 it is possible, through regular physical

> *We are always worrying about whether or not we are attractive to others. Attractiveness is not just about externalities. It's about how you feel inside and how well your body functions, how healthy you are. In all my years in the fitness industry, I've never seen a fit person who wasn't good-looking. If you're fit, you look good!*

activity, to get back the physique you had when you were 25. But at 45, as opposed to 25, you take longer to recover from exercise and you have to be more consistent about doing it. Whereas a 25-year-old can miss a week of exercise and not notice a difference, a 45-year-old will have to maintain a routine every other day. Long-term conditioning will accomplish a lot. In terms of looking good, regular exercise is going to help you look good a lot longer.

As you get older, you lose on average half a pound of muscle a year. If you stay fit you won't lose it, or you'll lose a lot less. By staying fit and strong, you also reduce your resting heart rate, which will give you a greater cardiovascular capacity than most people your age.

In this culture it's not realistic to think that you're not going to get caught in the "looking good" mindset.

Recognize that everyone thinks about it and you're not alone in that. But this doesn't mean you have to kill yourself over it. The thing to do is realize that everyone wants to look perfect, and then translate this goal to be the best that you can be.

Don't Make the Process Too Hard

WHEN I FIRST started in the fitness business in 1979, my background was as an athlete, and I had also experienced intense rehabilitation after my motorcycle accident. I thought the only way to exercise was "no pain, no gain." When people came to join my first club, I'd take them through the equipment and push them so hard that some of them would get sick. One day I hired a new accountant, Bill Shanks (who is still my accountant). At the time Bill was 29 and very fit — a basketball player. Whenever someone joined the club, I would call him or her two or three days later to see how it was going. Bill didn't come in for his second workout, so I phoned him. He said, "I can't get out of bed."

Here was this 29-year-old, very fit man and I had pushed him so hard that he couldn't get out of bed. I thought, "This isn't good," and I changed the whole strategy. When you push someone so hard that he or she collapses under the strain, this is called "training to failure." From that point on, I decided to train people only to success.

Now when we put a person on the equipment, we first look at her function. We want to make sure that she experiences the equipment with her whole range of motion. The number-one reason people get old is that they lose flexibility, so a full range of motion is important. We start them off with weights they can manage for the whole range of motion. Invariably most people can do more weight in a short range of motion, but only half the weight with a full range of motion. For example, you can easily lift a 20-pound box of groceries from your hips to your chest. But pick it up off the floor and put it over your head — that's a full range of motion, and it's much harder.

Another reason we want people to go through the whole range of motion is that you are less likely to get injured when you're strong. We know, for example, that 80 percent of back injuries are caused by weak muscles. Once people start doing exercises through their full range of motion, they can increase the weights really quickly.

What does this have to do with looking good? If you are exercising using your whole range of motion, within your first month you will start to build muscle. You'll gain two pounds of muscle in that first month. Every pound of muscle consumes 50 to 100 calories per day in order to maintain itself, so you've just taken your base metabolic rate up. You've increased your metabolism's need for food. Every time you lose a pound of muscle, your metabolic rate goes down 50 calories. As you get older, say from age 30 to 40, you'll lose ten pounds of muscle in that decade. So you'll have to consume considerably fewer calories in order to stay the same weight and not gain fat. But if you keep the same amount of muscle, you don't have to eat less. If you add on two pounds of muscle, you can actually eat more. And as you gain muscle, you'll look better.

Often a person who comes in to exercise says, "My weight hasn't changed." But what he has done is lose two pounds of fat and put on two pounds of muscle. Muscle takes up less space than fat and it looks better. If you have more muscle, you can consume more calories and not get fatter. That's why fit people tend to look better longer. You can eat more if you have muscle, and you have more energy because the muscle makes your life easier.

Looking good in terms of having more muscle gives you benefits far beyond just your appearance. There is less physical stress on the body. If you are capable of moving 100 pounds on a back machine and then you have to pick up 30 pounds of groceries, that's only 30 percent of what you are capable of. Your chances of getting injured are lower. The same thing happens with flexibility. If you're flexible enough to stretch to get a coffee cup from the top shelf of your cupboard, your life is less stressful. Or if your child grabs and pulls you, you won't pull a muscle if you're flexible and strong. Injuries happen when you're weaker.

Let's take another example — carpal tunnel syndrome. People get that from using computers all day. But if you strengthen your wrists and your hands, shoulders, arms, back, and chest, so all that weight isn't just on your wrists, then your risk of carpal tunnel syndrome will be drastically lower.

Statistics show that fit people live a minimum of two years longer than the average population. I believe it is much longer. But what statisticians don't talk about is quality of life. If you knew that you could dance 10 dances in a row and not be winded, wouldn't that be pleasurable? If you knew that you need never worry about what is in the grocery bag because you can lift it and not hurt yourself, wouldn't that make your life easier? All these things equip you to handle life. It makes a difference for the people you love, as well as in your work and in your play.

The Glow of Health and Well-Being

IF YOU GIVE your body a total fitness program — one that is easy to do — you're not going to put on more weight and you're going to have a lot more energy. Looking good becomes feeling good, and it leads to longevity and quality of life. If I could get only one message across in this chapter, it would be this: There are no rights or wrongs about looking good; there is only what's right for you and your body type. Don't look at someone else and decide she's "right" and you're "wrong." You'll find that, as you get fit, you become more accepting of your body. You'll start to look good because you'll radiate a confidence from within. You will have the glow of good health and well-being, and people will find that attractive.

I like to say that exercise is a form of self-respect. If you look after your own health, it means you're capable of being involved with others. Jimmy Buffett has a song about "people who have nothing to share, like driving around without a spare." If you're taxed physically and emotionally, you're driving around without a spare. You may have a "spare tire" of fat, but you won't have that extra energy and vitality.

The body is absolutely phenomenal. It can do wonders. Most people can achieve a fitness level they would never dream possible. Ninety-nine percent of people can do things they don't believe they can do. I didn't really get into skiing until I was 35 years old, and I had rheumatoid arthritis. I go helicopter skiing now, and I still have arthritis. You can do so much. A person who hasn't walked a block can be walking five miles six months later.

The body wants exercise so badly. It needs it, craves it, and it rewards you when you do it, by making you look good and feel good. There isn't anything you can spend your money on that does as much for you as exercise. There isn't a medication you can buy, or a car, or a house, or a trip that will make you feel the way you do when your body is fit and healthy.

As I said at the beginning of this chapter, most people start to exercise because of the way they look, but after six months or so, they stay with it because they feel good. Self-acceptance, self-awareness, and fitness are a circle. When that circle is complete and you're moving around it every day with a light, fit step, people will come up to you and say, "Wow! You look good!"

Here are some "Wow! Looking good!" people:

RICH BLASSER

IT'S NOT MY being overweight or underweight that stopped the progression. It was the distance between laziness and willpower. If only the future could be changed with minimal effort, my laziness could rule time. My minimal effort had cruelly proven to be a poor theory, as I could not see my toes in the shower any more. I would look at my stomach and be awestruck by its sheer magnificence — it was huge. I was not impressed. If I decided to trash my stomach, I was going to have to lift a finger — not my idea of overwhelming excitement, although I was not about to buy a back-up beeper for my big butt.

So — my brain decided to join GoodLife. My body decided not to join GoodLife. The two of them argued and argued over and over for I don't know how long. The two of them were really ticking me off.

I looked at the treadmill and thought, "I could do that," while my body was yelling, "Don't get me on that devil-made torture machine!" But I did, because I rarely listen to my body, and why should I? It doesn't know what it's doing anyway.

Then I looked at the weights and thought, "I could do that too." In time-stopping horror, my body was screaming, "Have you lost it? Are you insane? Don't you touch those things!" Once again, my brain won the war and I continued to disregard my body's request for freedom. The easy thing to do would be to quit, go home, lie on the couch, eat ice cream, and watch TV.

It's three years later, and I've continued to work out. I can see significant shrinkage — in my stomach, that is. The moral of the story: I don't know. You'll have to figure that out on your own. All I know is that I have more energy now, I'm stronger, and I feel better about myself. Now go away and do something!

AVRIL FARLAM

BIG — THAT WAS ME — bigger than I wanted to be for as long as I can remember. Not fat, not exactly. I could always carry a little more weight than some people because, on me, the weight did not all collect at my waist or my butt. It spread out everywhere. I had big arms, a big neck, and big thighs — I was just too big.

My diet seemed fine and when I tried fad diets I might lose a little weight. But soon it would be back. I seemed active enough. Heck, back in high school I even made the school basketball team.

Being big never really held me back. I just wished I could be smaller. I had a good marriage and a great family. I graduated from law school and built a busy law practice. I was the model superwoman with the world by the tail and an extra 25 pounds.

One day I was referred to a surgeon. She dealt with my health problem and then said I needed to start a comprehensive and disciplined program of regular exercise. I started to explain how that wouldn't be necessary, how active I was, how I wasn't really fat — I'd been big as long as I could remember. When I stopped talking, she explained how that wasn't the same as an overall workout that was available at the fitness centre she attended. She even offered to take me to her club and she introduced me to everyone there.

At first it was awful. I could only work out for a few minutes at a time and only at the lowest settings on the equipment. Tiny, 18-year-old girls, a little bigger than my daughter, and 60-year-old women, who could almost be my mother, could outshine me. It both embarrassed and inspired me. I never really knew I was in such bad shape.

Soon I could last a little longer and at higher levels. After a few weeks I went with my family for our regular bike ride. Instead of my husband and kids riding off into the distance and then stopping to wait for me, this time they stayed with me. Then it suddenly struck me that I was keeping up with them!

With my law practice I couldn't work out in the evenings consistently, so I learned to get up an hour earlier and exercise to start my day. Soon I wasn't tired anymore because I was sleeping better. I started to feel good for the first time in my life.

I got into a pretty consistent pattern of 20 to 25 workouts every month. I felt better and better. I often worked out with my doctor friend and she taught me things about nutrition and lifestyle. Even my husband and children became healthier.

As the weeks and months progressed, so did I. That first fall I was having a terrible time in my favourite stores finding clothes that fit properly, and I realized that I couldn't wear plus sizes any more. My husband cheerfully helped me mark and pin my old clothes and armloads of garments had to be taken in. He began to tell me that I looked great. I kept a pair of my old pants and tried them on every once in a while, just to marvel at the changes.

Working out became so enjoyable that I began to dread going on vacation because I would miss my exercise. I got really good at finding other clubs to use when I was out of town.

I had always thought it was normal to feel bad all the time, exhausted all the time. I always expected to die at a relatively young age like many of my relatives. Not anymore. The other night, as I was trying on some of my new, slim clothes in front of my new, full-length mirrors, my husband and I were talking about things we would do well into our retirement. I'm only in my forties, but the way I feel now, I expect to live forever.

When I look in the mirror now, I marvel at how my life has changed. Reflected back is not a big person. It's not me plus 25 pounds. It's not me dressing to look thinner. The reflection is just me. The small me I always wanted to be.

Just me. I like that.

ALBERT HOWELL

BEFORE I STARTED working out, I didn't have a lot of confidence.
Even though I'm fairly slim, I'm not very muscular. I was
intimidated by my feelings of inadequacy about my
body's shape. I joined GoodLife just to get some exercise, and since there are a lot of locations, I couldn't use
the "it's too far" excuse to avoid working out.

At first I was nervous about entering a "jock palace,"
but the staff and members were all friendly and I never
felt that I didn't belong. After a few weeks, a strange thing
happened. I felt better. I looked better. I felt sharper
mentally and my confidence started growing. Now I can
see myself with the kind of body I've only ever dreamed
of. I may never look like that in real life, but as long as I
keep working out, I know I'll stay healthy, confident, and
smart enough to know I don't need that kind of body to
be happy.

ERNIE ROBINSON

OVER THE PAST 10 years I have been an avid reader of self-improvement authors: Norman Vincent Peale, Dr. Robert Schuller, Dale Carnegie, and so forth. I would heartily recommend this route to those interested in improving their inner selves and human relations. Unfortunately my outer self — my body — was suffering from the "Dunlop disease": My stomach "done lopped" over my belt! Lethargy had replaced energy, which had done a number on my self-confidence. Potato chips were my best friend and my arteries were rebelling, giving me a stationary heartbeat of 96 beats per minute.

The program my fitness counsellor placed me on — cardio and muscle-building on alternate mornings — sent me off to work each day with the confidence that I had already done more exercise by 7:30 a.m. than most people do in a whole day. My sense of discipline — needed for early morning workouts — gives me a tremendous energy boost every single day. I find I can even "short-circuit" illness (flu and colds used to be common for me) by going to the club and charging through with some exercise that leaves me feeling invigorated instead of sick.

I am now proud to take off my shirt in the summertime. "Dunlop" is no longer a tire around my middle and I've brought my resting heart rate down by 20 beats (except when I look at my girlfriend!).

If you are young or old, avoid the "furniture disease" (where your chest drops into your drawers). There is a good life out there for all of us!

KAREN TRUSSLER

I COULD SAY it's the nine pounds I've lost, but it's more than that. It's improved health. It's the gentle motivation to keep going even when it's hard to find the time, much less the energy, to do one more move. It's the way my clothes fit. It's the energy I get from regular workouts. It's the opportunity to be self-caring and to find more stamina to do all the things I want to do. It's the promise of good health in old age.

JOHN OTA

EXERCISE DIDN'T CHANGE my life — it saved my life.

In 1995, when I turned 40, I took a good look at myself in the mirror and it wasn't a pretty picture. My untoned body and a Michelin tire around my waist were less than flattering for a man about to embark on the "best years of my life." An inconsistent diet and lack of exercise had led to arrhythmia and a heart murmur. With a history of heart problems on both sides of my family, I knew my sedentary lifestyle was leading me to an early cardiac arrest.

Midlife crisis can be handled in different ways. Some people buy fast cars. Others trade in for younger partners. I used a fortieth birthday present from my mother-in-law to join a GoodLife club. Already possessing an obsessive personality, I threw myself into a gradual but steady program of aerobics and weight training, with fitness checks every three months. Slowly, gradually, I could feel things changing for the better. With a drop in my body-fat level and a healthier diet, I began feeling stronger and gaining stamina, and, best of all, the arrhythmia and heart murmur disappeared.

Along the way a martial-arts course eventually led me to additional karate classes. And once my butt got hardened by the unyielding seat of the stationary bike, I started Power Pacing. With rivers of sweat pouring down my face, lungs hoovering up oxygen, and legs whirling to the wails of Madonna, my mind and body found a way to escape completely the tension of the office.

Besides a physical improvement, going to the club set off a number of processes that enhanced my life in a holistic way. Professionally, my noon-hour workouts are also a change of scenery from the workplace, which actually increases my productivity and gives some perspective to my life. In addition, I was fortunate to meet people at the club who, through their own backgrounds, have given me advice and enriched my professional life.

Emotionally, the opportunity to release pent-up energy in a positive atmosphere puts me in a better mood all day. Like the eye of a storm, my workout is the calm and balance of my frantic day.

The bad news is that, after all this, I'll never be asked to pose in a Calvin Klein underwear ad. The good news is that my body and mind are in better condition than at any other time of my life. Without exercise, I had stress, tension, and arrhythmia. With exercise, I have a fit body, a positive attitude, and the promise of a longer life. I also feel that I've done everything I can to shut the door on that potential heart attack. Physically, emotionally, and professionally, my life is a thousand percent better than before I started exercising four years ago. It all starts with my fitness.

CHAPTER THREE

FEELING GOOD

THE REASON PEOPLE keep exercising — the reason people like to be fit — is really only partially about how they look. This is perhaps only 25 percent of the equation, even though looking good, as we've been talking about it, is often the primary motivator to get them exercising in the first place. Seventy-five percent of the equation is how they feel. The best way to describe it is to refer to the lack of feeling good. An athlete, or someone else who has always been active, will say, "Do you remember how it felt so good when we scored that touchdown / won that race / painted the whole house in one day?" and so forth. But a person who has never been fit doesn't have that memory of "how it felt so good."

If I asked, "Have you ever had the flu?" most people would say yes. What was it like? They would probably answer, "I felt terrible. I had low energy. I had such aches and pains." Well, that's what it's like being unfit. But, unlike the flu, it doesn't just hit you out of the blue. "Unfitness" happens slowly, insidiously, so you don't really notice.

Let's take alcohol consumption as an example. The first time you get drunk the hangover feels terrible. You do it for a week, and it feels really terrible. You do it for a year, and it's "the way life is." You habituate to feeling bad, and you think that's normal. Your functional level is like a hangover. It's an "unfit-over." Your body knows it should have energy and vitality, but your brain learns to accept a lower quality of life.

Imagine that you have had allergies all your life and your nose is always stuffed up. Then imagine that one day, all of a sudden, you wake up and you don't have the sniffles anymore — you can breathe. You can smell that apple pie baking. You can smell the lilac bushes. That's what being fit is like. For a fit person, the sun is shining. You go to the store and you have extra energy. You talk to someone and you have extra enthusiasm. That's feeling good. It didn't happen because you sat and read a couple of books on self-esteem. It happened because your body is functioning as it should be, and this puts you — body, mind, and soul — into a state of well-being.

If your fitness levels starts to decline into unfitness, you keep noticing things you can't do. Then you become

You are the hero of your own life. Give yourself credit for all your efforts to become fit and healthy. The fact that you get up every day and participate in fitness activities, and that you've chosen not to be just a spectator — that makes you a hero. Acknowledge yourself for that.

wrapped up in not wanting to do something that would expose your weakness. You don't go swimming because you don't want people to see your belly. You don't play squash because you get winded. The fun that you would get from water skiing, or hiking, or playing with your grandchildren, or running with your dog — all that is part of feeling good. You can't run around with your dog or your kids if your low energy levels have got you slouching on the couch.

When you exercise for 20 minutes three times a week, suddenly life becomes so much "tastier." There is a chemical reaction in your body that tells you physical activity is the right thing to do. You don't need to know the biochemistry of endorphins to know that they make you feel good and that they are triggered by exercise. And exercising is unbelievably easy. All you need to do, three times a week, is raise your heart rate enough so that when you're talking, you're gasping a little bit for breath — not choking for breath, just gasping. All you need to do, three times a week, is make your muscles a little stronger than they were, by means of what we call a progressive overload system. You'll notice within six weeks how much better you feel.

Isn't Exercise Boring?

MOST PEOPLE FEEL better right away for one huge reason — self-control. They have taken control of their bodies. If you just relax and listen to your body, it will tell you what it needs in order to feel good. But, you may ask, what about the fact that — after six weeks or six months — exercise becomes routine, or you lose motivation?

When people say they get tired of exercise, there are two reasons. One is that you have gone beyond "enough is enough" and just push and push until you can't push any more. The other reason is a feeling of boredom. You ask, "How can I run the same route three times a week? How can I run on a treadmill? How can I lift the same weights?"

In answer to that I say that we are very lucky. If you do your activity outside, nature makes it such a wonderful place. People on the street or in the park are wonderful to see. Wherever you are, you can find delight in your surroundings. See that half hour three times a week as a time to become mindful of and alive to your surroundings. If you're lucky enough to go to a club that has different facilities, the equipment is so space-age and computerized that most people are fascinated by it. The machines tell you what your heart rate is and how fast you're going. They tell you how you did last week or last month. A lot of fitness clubs have TVs you can watch while you're exercising. You can read while you ride a stationary bicycle, and lots of people read when they're on a StairMaster.

But what I try to get people to do is — nothing. Just let your brain float and be aware of whatever thoughts float into your mind and out again. That's what happens in meditation. In meditation you clear the mind and let it float. Exercise can be a form of moving meditation. In giving yourself a little "me" time, you can turn your attention inward while you're exercising, and lower your stress level. Many people these days practise sitting meditation to relax and reduce stress. You can bring this same mind state to your exercising.

Separate Exercise and Sport

ANOTHER ISSUE HAS an impact on feeling good about exercising. Most people have a mental "failure syndrome" created by the experience of not being successful at school in basketball, volleyball, track and field, or other sports. The key to feeling good in exercise is to separate exercise from sport. When we were at school, physical education was often about being the best athlete, and those of us who weren't good athletes felt like failures. No one patted us on the back and said "good for showing up." It's still that way in school physical education programs. The emphasis in many schools is still on athleticism and not on fitness. Our schools continue to breed failure into generations of couch-potato kids because, let's face it, very few of us are going to become good athletes. As adults we still carry this fear of embarrassment, this shame we felt at not being very good at sports, this fear of being laughed at, and so we avoid going to a fitness club. We avoid exercise.

Fitness Doesn't Require Skill

WHEN YOU GET to the point where you do decide to go to a fitness club or buy a piece of exercise equipment, or you resolve to take a brisk walk every evening, give yourself a big round of applause for just showing up in your own life and taking control. Next, realize that the activities you need for fitness are non-athletic. They do not require skill. Not one activity you need to do for fitness requires special skill. If you can hold a pen, if you can brush your teeth, if you can open a book, you can do fitness activities.

The simplest form of exercise is walking. Almost everyone can walk (unless you have a disability that makes walking impossible). If you went for a walk on a regular basis for half an hour, five times a week, you would be a lot fitter than most of your friends and colleagues, just from doing that. It would help your arteries, lower your fatty acids, help with your blood pressure, and help control your weight.

If you want to help your heart as well, you need to go further and do activity that gets your heart rate up into what we call the training zone, three times a week, for 12 to 20 minutes. You can do that by walking really fast. You can do it by jogging. You can ride a stationary

> *Understand that in fitness, being "good" means achieving your own personal best, not being better than others. Every step you take toward improving the health and fitness of your body is a personal triumph.*

bicycle at home or at a club. This requires no learning curve. If you have two legs that can move, we can put you on a bicycle and you will know how to do it. You can do the same thing by walking on a treadmill or using a piece of equipment called a cross-trainer. You can learn how to use a cross-trainer in less than five minutes. Some equipment may have a longer learning curve, perhaps half an hour, but none of it is rocket science in terms of learning how to use it.

For strength training, you can be taught how to do a push-up in two minutes and a sit-up in one minute. If you go to a club, most of them have strength-training equipment where all you have to do is move pins to change the weight. You can learn to use the computerized strength-training machines in less than half an hour. Fitness facilities have nothing to do with being athletic. Of course you may see athletes at fitness clubs, or you may use fitness in order to become athletic, if that is what you want to do. Some people do use exercise as training for specific sports. But fitness stands alone, quite distinct from sports. Fitness is mostly about making your body function the way it was intended to, so that your brain functions the way it was intended to, so that you get the most and the best out of life.

It's So Easy

THE PROBLEM IS that we take our bodies for granted. We just
assume that we will be healthy and that we don't have to
do anything to guarantee that we stay healthy. But when
we get sick or have an accident, we realize we can't take
our bodies for granted. Sometimes it is sickness or adver-
sity that brings us to the pursuit of fitness (we'll be talking about that later in this book).

The reality is that, in terms of our fitness and
health, we're born with the opportunity to be everything
we can be. Over thousands of years of evolution, Nature
has made it easy to do what it takes in order to feel good.
You have 168 hours in a week. Your body will function
fantastically if you devote an hour and a half to two
hours of that 168 to your fitness. Two hours a week is
104 hours a year — 4.3 days — spent on exercise.
Assuming that the average person lives 78 years, 335
days of your life would be devoted to exercise. It's been
proven that you gain two years or more if you exercise
regularly. Let's assume that you get 10 or 15 more years
of longevity from doing fitness activities on a regular
basis throughout your adult life. Think of the payoff. At
the least, it's more than 100 percent. No other investment you can make will give you that.

People often ask me, "If all this is true, then why in

our culture are most people so abysmally unfit?" We have to consider that the "unfitness epidemic," with its chronic anxiety, fatigue, and feelings of unease, is really only a blip on the human radar screen of history. It's only been about 50 years since people didn't have to do something physical every day. The ease of life we have today in the Western world is relatively recent. Our evolutionary concept of needing physical activity hasn't caught up. Twenty percent of the population is aware and does physical activity. The other 80 percent knows, but is not doing it. Nine percent of the total population of the United States and Canada is working out at fitness clubs. This percentage is gradually rising by 1 to 2 percent a year.

We used to get so much exercise in times past that it wore us out. We would die young from years of 16-hour

My favourite "feel good" fitness activities:
I love to rollerblade. I find the feeling of speed exhilarating, and rollerblading is a non-impact activity. I love biking, especially where there are lots of beautiful trees, fresh air, and sunshine. Swimming, climbing, and skiing are also favourites of mine.

days in the coal mines or in the fields. That's not the case today. Now we have to exercise so as not to rust out from inactivity. Work has changed to become less physically challenging but more mentally stressful. I think a time is coming when more people will become smart enough to realize that this is what they have to do, especially when they discover that it doesn't have to be hard — that it's actually very easy. It's actually fun.

Think about eating. You know that you need to eat. The gnawing in your stomach when you're hungry tells you that. And if you don't eat for a few weeks, you die. What happens when you don't exercise is that you're hastening your death, but your death is "making haste slowly." And while you're hastening your death, you're lowering your quality of life because you'll be more tired and feel less vital.

To get people to the state of looking good and feeling good, we in the fitness industry have to find ways to take the fear out of exercise. The images of perfection and athleticism in fitness have to go. These images have become prevalent in our society because extremes attract attention. It's not newsworthy to show a picture of a hundred women who have two children and who are all within 10 percent of their ideal body weights, comfortable with themselves, and looking fine. But if I show you the most overweight person in the world, that will get in the news. Or if I show you the fittest, most toned body in the world, people will say, "Wow, look at that."

Magazines and TV make money from promoting perfection. They will tell you there are a thousand different ways to strengthen your biceps. It's not that complicated. It's the same thing as telling you a thousand ways to turn the steering wheel of your car. Once you do it, it's really easy. You don't need to know a thousand different ways; you only need to know one or two. Fitness is the same. The most complicated pieces of equipment in a gym are barbells and dumbbells. You don't need to use them. Most of the consumer magazines put emphasis on them, but you never have to touch one. Even if you decide you want to use these weights, someone can teach you in six easy sessions.

Even fitness classes are designed so that anyone can just do them. There are advanced classes that are more complicated, but you don't need to go to them to get fit. People go for the challenge. You'll get fit whether or not you take up the challenge of higher-skill classes. It's also true that some people will join a fitness club, start becoming fit, and then discover they have some athletic talent. So they run marathons, perfect their golf

> *Doing enjoyable fitness activities in a natural setting has an added bonus: the scenery itself gives off lots of positive energy. I find that being in a setting like that is almost meditative. Most of my "meditation" is active. It's impossible to be high up in the mountains and not feel spiritual.*

games, or win squash games. But that's not everybody, and it doesn't have to be you.

If the statistics continue to indicate that 80 percent of people don't participate in exercise, I can foresee that our longevity as a nation may decrease by a couple of years. We'll begin to pay the price for our lack of activity. On the other hand, if we can move from 20 percent of the population participating in exercise to 40 percent, that will create an enormous jump in positive health outcomes. If things continue as they are now I see a huge gap, between overweight people dying younger, with a greater cost to the health and social systems, and the ones who are carrying those costs and getting mad about it. There is a backlash now against smokers. They have more sick days, are less productive, and die sooner, and in the process of dying they cost the health system more. Non-smokers now outnumber smokers and there is mounting pressure to combat nicotine addiction further. Ten or 30 years down the road we may see the same backlash against lazy, inactive people.

But let's get back to feeling good. What other things can we say about feeling good through fitness? Even sex is better if you're fit. Your body looks better. It turns on your partner more. You feel better to touch. You have the physical capability to last longer and enjoy yourself. You're not going to have a heart attack or pull a muscle in the process. It's fun. It feels good.

Exercise also has positive effects on depression. Studies have shown that exercise elevates mood. A lot of emotional problems are caused by feelings of loss of control. If you feel in control, you feel better about yourself. And the first step toward gaining control is doing what you know innately is right — physical activity.

Feeling good is an intangible that, paradoxically, is tangible. It's hard to describe in exact words, but you know it when you feel it. You can't bottle it. You can't save it. You can't store it. It's like a smile — it's just there.

Here are some people who have discovered the inner treasure of feeling good:

KATHRYN MCEWIN

EXACTLY ONE YEAR ago I decided to rearrange the priorities in my life. Becoming more healthy and feeling healthier were right near the top of the list. So off I went on the quest for a gym that could help me reach my goal of becoming healthier. When I walked through the door of the GoodLife club in my community, I knew I had found the right place. The equipment is top-notch, the staff are friendly, encouraging, and supportive, and they never forget your name. They set me up on a great program that combined cardio, weight training, and stretching. Before long I could not only see the results of exercise when I looked in the mirror but I could feel the results inside. My confidence started to increase, my energy perked up, my endurance increased, and I felt so good!

If I could give anyone advice about exercise, it would be to stick with it and you will see and feel great results. Sometimes it's a struggle to find the time to become healthier, but once you make it a priority, you find time for exercise. In one year I have lost 20 pounds and 9.5 inches, and my resting heart rate has dropped 16 beats. My body-fat percentage has also decreased by 13 percent. To get these results, I exercised more and ate healthier. I can now fit into clothes I haven't been able to wear since my college years. But most important, I feel great!

BRENDA PAUL

I FIND THAT working out at the gym is imperative for me. I try to go to the gym at least two or three times a week. Working out for me is good for my emotional, physical, spiritual, and mental well-being. I feel better, I look better, and I have added energy. When I feel good, I go to the gym to work on myself physically. When I feel a little down, I go to the gym to work off stress and tensions. I have also gone to the gym for serenity. I find sometimes I can work on my body and detach myself from all outside negativity and pressures of the day. At times it can actually be a form of meditation for me. As I grow older, I also notice that I can control the aches and pains that I experience when I am not staying as active. I know how necessary this is for my self-confidence as well.

I am 48 years old, a single mother of two children, ages 19 and 21. My children tell me how proud they are to have a mother as fit and attractive as I have kept myself. I find I am in much better shape than many other people in my age group. I am also proud of myself for the personal motivation and incentive to work for this personal goal. I hope through all my hard work that I will be able to slow down the aging process in order to always be able to enjoy the happiness of this wonderful life.

MARGIE MASTELLAR

I AM 72 and I am sure that going to a fitness club keeps me young, healthy, and fit. I have lost inches and pounds, and I have gained many new friends. All my life I have enjoyed all sorts of sports — swimming, rowing, biking, and aerobics. So when my friends say, "At our age, we don't need it anymore," I answer, "At our age we need it twice as much." My bone density test said I have the bones of a young adult. Doing the weight training keeps them strong. I feel wonderful.

LYNNE MCDONALD

I WOKE UP one day, after a few hectic years of raising three young sons, to find I had a low energy level, poor sleeping patterns, falling self-esteem because my clothes were not fitting the way I swear they did the week before, and increased irritability from coping with a full-time job and a growing, active family.

I had faithfully worked out with weights and performed cardiovascular activities three times a week for years. However, I had fallen into the trap of not challenging myself and trying new things. I was determined to see changes in my body composition and cardiovascular endurance, and in turn see positive changes to my general appearance, self-esteem, stress-coping abilities, and eating habits.

With the assistance and encouragement of GoodLife staff and a personal trainer, my lifestyle changed dramatically. My experience has given me a better understanding of the importance of resistance training with cardiovascular activity, increased awareness of how food fuels your body and a reminder of the importance of goal-setting and just plain having fun.

My body fat has decreased considerably. I have copious amounts of energy, to the point that my kids cannot keep up with me. I have also had co-workers comment that I am much calmer and more relaxed in dealing with daily issues.

I've reached all my original goals and continue to set new, challenging ones. A desire to inform others of the benefits of physical activity, resistance training, and well-balanced eating habits led me to become certified as a personal trainer. I love this part of my life, to the point that I don't consider it work!

CHAPTER FOUR

A GOOD
WEIGHT

Everyone talks about having a "perfect weight." Weight is an obsession in this culture because we have tied it to our sense of selfhood and self-esteem. People will go to great lengths to "do something" about their weight. What do people mean when they say they want the perfect weight? They mean that when you walk down the street, people will stop to cast admiring glances your way; that every photographer in the world will want to put you on the cover of *Vogue* or *GQ* magazine; that every one of your friends will be jealous and wish he or she could look like you.

Wait a second. It's not going to happen. You will never make yourself happy with someone else's opinion of what your weight should be. All those criteria of weight I've just mentioned are based on someone else's opinion. You need to decide what your weight should be, a weight that takes into account your body type and lifestyle, the weight that will make you happy.

When it comes to weight, the influence of public media is insidious. Several times in this book you will find me saying that we must be wary of the images of perfection we see in magazines, on TV, and in the movies. Ninety-nine percent of the population simply cannot look like those models and celebrities. In fact, very often when you see a model or movie star in person, you find he or she doesn't look nearly so perfect in the flesh as on the page or the screen.

Oftentimes we find ourselves buying into the obsession with perpetual thinness that is the current cultural ideal, often with very negative results for our health and self-esteem. We lose sight of the fact that different periods of history have had differing images of attractiveness. Some eras have valued the full-figured body, just as our era seems to be going to extremes with thinness. We need to learn to distinguish between a good weight, which is possible for us, and a perfect weight, which doesn't exist. We need to know the difference between a good weight and overweight. We need to understand that our body weight is an aspect of our total overall health, and that our ideal weight is the weight we are when our bodies are functioning at their best.

What Is a Good Weight?

THE RIGHT WEIGHT for you as an individual depends on a number of factors. First of all, take into consideration your role in life. Are you a competitive athlete? Competitive athletes make up only a small percentage of the total population. Let's assume that only 2 percent of people could be classified as such. Competitive athletes need to have lower body fat so that they can move faster. If you are one, then you're likely doing training and understand your diet patterns well enough that body weight is a non-issue. So most competitive athletes will have a good weight that is determined by their sports, how they train, and how they compete.

Many more people in the population are recreational athletes, taking up sports for fun and pleasure, and maybe mild competition as well. For recreational athletes, a man's body weight should be 10 to 20 percent fat, and a woman's should be between 15 and 25 percent fat, depending on whether he or she is an ectomorph, endomorph, or mesomorph. These body-fat percentages are good guidelines, even if you're not a recreational athlete.

Most people are not athletes, recreational or otherwise. In fact, as I've been saying, the pursuit of fitness is something quite separate from athleticism. So let's look at body fat for the average population. In this society there are many people who have more than 30 percent body fat. Forty percent body fat is considered obese. If you have more than 30 percent body fat, you're distinctly overweight. This is unhealthy — it's going to reduce how long you live, and it's going to cut down on the quality of your life every single day.

Rather than reading charts that say if you're such and such a height, your weight should be x, it's far better to use body-fat percentage as your guideline. No matter what your height or your bone structure, if the percentage of total body fat falls within an acceptable range, you will be a good weight. If you are a male and you have 10 to 15 percent body fat, you should be happy with that. That's a really good weight. You wouldn't want to weigh less than that, and there's no need to. If you are a woman and you have around 20 to 25 percent body fat, that's a good weight for most women. If you are a female with less than 15 percent body fat, you will tend to lose your menstrual cycle, which isn't a healthy thing to have happen. You should weigh within these parameters of body fat, between 10 and 30 percent, which is a pretty flexible range that allows for all kinds of body types. In reality, for most people, it's between 15 and 25 percent.

I would tell a man that if he reaches 20 percent

body fat, he should be thinking about increasing exercise and decreasing his intake of calories — now, before it gets ahead of him. I would tell a woman that if she reaches 30 percent body fat, she needs to increase exercise and decrease her caloric intake — now, before it gets ahead of her. So if you weigh 150 pounds and 40 percent of your weight is body fat, you are overweight. But if you weigh 200 pounds and 15 percent of your weight is body fat, you are not overweight. The variation between 10 and 30 percent takes into account your body type (ectomorph, endomorph, or mesomorph), whether you're male or female, the age and stage of life you are at, the stress level you might be experiencing, whether you're competitive or more laid-back, how active you are, and so forth. Once you drop below 10 percent body fat, you are underfed (unless you are a high-level athlete). You're not getting enough nutrition. This condition affects only a small percentage of the population. By far the majority of us are overfed.

Body fat can be measured with fat calipers or with bio-impedance testing. These methods can measure how much water is in your body, how much bone, how much muscle, and so forth. A bio-impedance machine costs several thousand dollars and some fitness clubs have them. Good calipers cost about $600, and many clubs use them. A well-trained and qualified fitness professional can help you determine the ratio of body fat in your overall weight.

The tests take only about five or 10 minutes. The feedback from the tests takes longer than the actual tests, because most of us are distressed at first to discover that we're carrying too much body fat. But this is the starting point from which you can begin to make healthy decisions to do something about your excess fat. Even if you don't take fat-measurement tests, your mirror is a good gauge. If you look at your naked body in the mirror and there's two or three inches of fat hanging over your waist, it's likely that you have too much body fat.

Factor in Eating

EXERCISE PLAYS A crucial role in weight control, but eating patterns must also be factored in. It's possible to be fit and fat. You can exercise like crazy and still be eating way too much. For example, when I ran the Boston Marathon in 1981, I weighed 225 pounds. During the years that I rowed, I weighed between 200 and 210. I rowed four hours a day, which is not what most of the population would do. But when I ran, it was only three times a week. I ran hard and long so that my body would adjust to running the distance. But I also ate way too much, so that in the process of training for the marathon I gained 15 pounds. It's not just how much you eat, it's also the quality of your food. Eating protein, complex carbohydrates, fruits, and vegetables makes infinitely more sense than ingesting fats, such as greasy french fries. We all know this, but we so easily "forget."

Sometimes we may think a person is at a good weight, but his or her appearance is deceiving. There are some people who look really slim but who are tremendously unfit and weak. All they're doing is not eating. Then there are people with phenomenally low metabolisms who have trouble losing any weight at all, no matter what they do in terms of nutrition. And there are people with high metabolisms who have trouble keeping weight on. For people with extremely low and high metabolisms, professional help is often needed to help them adjust their weight in a positive direction.

But the majority of us are somewhere in the middle: normal metabolisms, eating too much, but not enough of the right foods, and not getting enough exercise. We all want to know what the good weight for us is and how to get there. You know when you feel good. Your body

---

Some of my favourite foods:

• *I don't drink coffee or tea, but I do love hot chocolate — in fact, anything chocolate. I call chocolate my fifth main food group. It's my motivator and reward.*

• *I love peanut butter, especially on a cinnamon bagel.*

• *Stir-fried entrees really appeal to me — especially a stir-fry with squash, turnip, and sweet potatoes.*

• *I really enjoy pineapple.*

• *I tried being a vegetarian once, but it didn't work for me. I do eat some red meat, but not that often. When I eat meat, it is most often chicken or seafood.*

• *My favourite meal of all: my mother's hamburgers!*

---

knows when it feels healthy and vital. You look in the mirror and you see a body that's healthy and functioning well and looks good both in and out of clothes. If that's what you see, chances are you're the right weight for you. You can achieve 95 percent of what you want for your weight simply by participating in the type of fitness routine I have been talking about in this book — three times a week, for 20 minutes to half an hour.

The reason most people start exercising is to lose weight. And indeed, exercise will help you lose weight in time. It doesn't happen overnight. This is a very important point, for most of us want instant results. At first when you start exercising, you will most likely put weight on, because in the first month or two you will gain three to four pounds of muscle. Muscle weighs more than fat for the area it takes up. A 130-pound woman may say after four weeks of exercise, "Look, I've put on four pounds and now weigh 134. What's going on?"

That's when I would say to her, "Don't your sweaters and pants fit looser? Don't you feel more toned? Don't you have more energy? Don't you feel good about yourself?" The initial weight gain in muscle will eventually translate into an overall reduction of body fat. As you lose the body fat and replace it with muscle, your weight will gradually adjust to where it should be for you to have a healthy, vital, and good-looking body. Trust the process and be patient. It works.

I never encourage people to modify their weights by not eating or only by restricting their diets. If you want to achieve weight control, you need a process of strength training and exercise combined with sensible eating. If you are simply not eating, you won't be getting enough vitamins and other nutrients. You will be on a constant seesaw between how much you eat versus how you look, and you will never be happy.

Why Dieting Doesn't Work

DIETING IS A way of training your body to cope with starvation mode. When you restrict your caloric intake to below what your body needs to feel satisfied, it thinks you're living five thousand years ago, when maybe the crops had failed or the hunters came back empty-handed. When the body senses starvation, it stores as much as it can as fat. Evolutionary biology has trained us to do that very efficiently.

At the same time, the body will break down muscles in order to get protein and energy, and as a result you get weaker. Remember that every pound of muscle uses 50 to 100 calories a day. When you break down a pound of muscle in the course of dieting, you will look as if you're losing weight. But you won't understand why your body doesn't look that much better and why you don't feel that much better. It's the opposite when you start exercising. Initially you put on some weight, but it's muscle. In the long run, exercise will help you lose fat and keep it off, and in the short run, you'll look and feel better.

In the case of losing muscle through dieting, if you lose five pounds of muscle, you've lost the ability to use 250 to 400 calories of your daily intake. So any time you go off the diet and begin eating as much as you used to, you'll quickly start to gain weight again. In addition, because you don't have the muscle you had before, you'll put weight on faster than you did before you dieted.

When you're on a diet that gives you fewer calories than you need, the body reacts as though it's threatened with starvation. So it will do what it knows it should do: It will push you to eat. That's why when you're on a diet you will often get food cravings, feel an increase in appetite, and fall off the wagon. You have to be superhuman to control your hunger.

A further problem is that our bodies also assume that we will engage in physical activity to build muscle back up, because for thousands of years that's exactly what we did. In the last 50 years we've seen the rise of the sedentary society. In the past we had to plant crops, run across fields, lift logs to make our houses, battle the elements. Today we can just go back to our computer terminals or turn on the TV. Our bodies don't put on muscle from day-to-day living anymore. So if you've lost weight by dieting, or if you've been sick, you should work with weights, circuit-train, build up your strength. It's the only way to rebuild muscle. The way to really lose weight and keep it off is to do strength training while you control your eating patterns.

Controlling
Your Eating

THERE IS A difference between dieting and controlling your eating. Dieting is just an across-the-board reduction of the number of calories you take in, often without regard for your body type, lifestyle, or activity level. Controlling your eating, on the other hand, involves saying to yourself something like, "For normal function I need three thousand calories. I need these calories from different types of food: for example, a third from protein, a third from carbohydrates, and a third from fruits and vegetables." This is very different from just cutting back.

Humans are omnivores. We need a balance of different types of food. Even vegetarian animals consume different types of plants. The majority of species survive by having variety in their diets. The coyote, which can survive in literally all environments, including cities and towns, will eat anything.

Controlling your eating means taking in the calories you need through the right balance of nutrition from the different food groups. It means making wise choices: for example, choosing a baked potato over french fries, or oil-and-vinegar dressing on your salad over creamy ranch dressing. Generally a woman needs about 2,500 calories a day and a man 3,500. There are some variations, depending on your age, size, and level of activity. But there are very few people who can satisfy their bodies' natural hunger with fewer than a thousand calories per day. So if you go on a diet of a thousand calories or less, you know you're getting less than half the normal intake you need. You're going to lose a lot of muscle. Furthermore, the body will take that thousand calories and convert it to fat. It will break down your biceps, quadriceps, and back muscles in order to get energy.

When you control your eating patterns within the proper number of calories for your lifestyle and body type, and you strength-train, you're going to get a much more desirable result. If you are controlling your eating patterns, but don't strength-train as well, up to 80 percent of what you eventually lose will be muscle. If you do strength-train, almost everything you burn off will be fat, and the food you take in will be used to build muscle. The key to a good weight is to eat within your normal caloric range and to exercise, incorporating strength training into your routine.

One of the misconceptions about exercise and weight control is that you need to do a lot of cardiovascular training to burn calories. Cardiovascular exercises do burn calories — while you're exercising. But if you build muscle, you're burning calories all the time. You need cardiovascular exercise to improve your heart and lungs, to get your whole "pipe system" working better, but to burn calories you have to keep doing it. If, on the other hand, you've added muscle, you don't have to eat less to burn off the calories. In cardiovascular fitness, you'll lose 10 percent of your cardiovascular efficiency if you miss a week of the exercises. With muscle, it goes away much more slowly; if you built muscle over six months, it would take that long for it to go away. If for some reason you miss some strength training, for example, if you're ill or on vacation, you have more of a "cushion" of strength. You will be able to regain strength quite readily when you re-start the exercises.

To me, achieving a good weight is not about denying yourself food. It's about balance. In fact, weight control shouldn't be painful. It should include enough leeway to allow occasional indulgence in your pet "not good for you" food group. In my case, that's chocolate. For some it might be a cold beer, or a hamburger with all the trimmings. You should never see achieving a good weight as a path of deprivation. It doesn't have to be. You can design your weight-control program to allow for a few perks.

Many people seek out professional weight-control programs from companies that claim to guarantee a certain level of weight loss within a certain length of time.

Any weight-control group or program that doesn't encourage exercise is not telling the whole story. Any weight-control program that encourages extremes of caloric reduction, or advocates ingesting great amounts of one particular food (for example, bananas or pine-apples) to the exclusion of others should be avoided. Any weight-control group that encourages exercise along with a balanced diet and that doesn't encourage extremes is OK. I think the best of these programs are those that teach us to make healthy choices, so that we can continue on our own.

Exercise Influences Appetite

FOR MOST PEOPLE, exercise will help balance appetite. For some, exercise may act as an appetite suppressant, but this does not hold for everyone, nor is it consistent. I think the most far-reaching effect of exercise on appetite lies in the psychological aspects of our makeup. A lot of us eat as a way to cope with stress. As children we learned that when we fell down and hurt ourselves, Mom would give us candy or a cookie to help us feel better. The idea was ingrained in many of us that eating makes us feel better emotionally. Often exercise will control the urge to eat because of its positive effect on stress levels. Exercise helps us feel less stress, so by extension it reduces the artificially created need to eat so as not to feel sad or stressed out.

Exercise also stabilizes your blood-sugar levels, and in this way helps you avoid the ups and downs of blood sugar that may cause you to want to eat. Then there is what I call the ripple effect of exercising on eating. You decide that you will exercise. You do it and it feels good. In the back of your mind is the thought, "I have just exercised. I need to be a little smarter about what I eat." The self-control you achieve through exercise extends to other areas of your life and helps give you the resolve you need to carry through with healthy lifestyle decisions.

Exercise and proper nutrition together help your body become a self-regulating system that will find its own wisdom for health within. Exercise and good nutrition support how your body is designed to work. Something that's running the way it's supposed to likes being that way. When you see a horse galloping in the pasture, you can tell that it loves to run. You just know. You don't need to prove it — you can see it in the flex and stretch of its sleek muscles and the speed and grace of its movements. It's the same for people. When you exercise and it feels good, and when you eat healthily and it feels good, you know that it feels good, that it's right.

Trust your body to tell you what's good. All you have to do is listen. We're really good at hearing the negative messages from our bodies, but not so good at paying attention to the positive ones. For example, if you bang your leg on a table and get a bruise, your body will register "ouch," and you will think, "This is bad. This is distressing." Think of it the other way around. You're exercising and eating well and your body sends you signals that say, "My blood is circulating freely. My skin looks better. My vision is clearer. I have more energy. It's easier to stand straight. I find things aren't bugging me as much. My stress level is lower." These signals are telling you that you are doing what you are supposed to do.

If you pay attention to your body, you'll eventually, instinctively know how much food you need and how much activity your body needs. In this culture, we have to re-learn these instincts, because we've lost touch with the intuitive health wisdom within us. That's why I think that nutrition and exercise experts, who have been well trained and who understand the need for balance and avoiding extremes, are very useful to have around. Ultimately, though, you can become your own expert. Give your body what it needs in terms of physical activity and balanced nutrition, and you will be rewarded with a good weight that you'll find easy to maintain, and you'll wake up every morning happy with the way you are.

Some of the many people who have found that a good weight is part of the good life:

CASSANDRA DAIGNEAULT

MY ENTIRE LIFE has been a struggle with obesity. Even as a young child I can remember being self-conscious and embarrassed by my weight. As I grew older, the problems escalated. I tried all the fad diets without success and eventually resigned myself to being fat forever. In 1997 my weight reached an all-time high of 290 pounds. As a registered nurse I understood the consequences of my excessive weight and feared for my health. Day-to-day activities had become a struggle. I became short of breath with minimal exertion and my legs and hips ached constantly. I worried continuously about things most people take for granted — Would I be able to find clothes that fit me? Would I fit into the seat at the theatre? Were people laughing at me? I felt like my entire life was out of control. Finally, in June of 1997, I faced a health crisis that made me realize that I had to take control of my weight. I joined GoodLife Fitness Clubs the next day, and my life has changed completely.

The trainers at the gym immediately put me at ease and made me realize that I was not alone in my battle of the bulge. Every six weeks I met with a personal trainer who helped me design an exercise program specific to my needs. Within weeks I began to see results. The pounds started to drop and I noticed a slow but steady increase in my energy level and stamina. As the months progressed, I was literally able to watch my body transform. Muscle replaced fat and my entire appearance began to change. I was elated each time I was able to move down a dress size. The regular program checks motivated me to stay on track and push myself a little harder. And on the occasions when my spirits lagged or I felt defeated, there was always someone there to address my concerns and get me back on track. Within a year I was less than 10 pounds away from my target weight of 160 pounds. Finally, on July 27, 1998, I reached my goal!

I have continued to set new goals and exercise is now an integral part of my life. I feel that my weight is now under my control rather than in control of me. I am healthier and happier than I have ever been and I am no longer ashamed and embarrassed by my body.

Since my weight loss I enjoy a much more active lifestyle. The increase in my level of confidence and self-esteem has helped me to form many new and healthy relationships. I even credit GoodLife for giving me the emotional well-being that led me to the man I am about to marry. Despite the occasional setback, I know that I will never go back to the unhealthy lifestyle I once lived.

DAVID TOZER

BY BECOMING INVOLVED with fitness, I was able to achieve goals that had eluded me for years. Like most people, I had put on some undesirable weight over the years and my blood pressure was up a little. I had tried a variety of programs to lose the weight, but nothing really worked. Using the GoodLife method, I was able to lose weight, increase my muscle strength, and lower my blood pressure.

I saw advertisements for the six-week weight-loss program at the club and decided to give it a try. I lost the weight the ad said I would lose. In particular, as the fat was lost, my clothes became noticeably looser. My waist size went down to a level it has not been in 20 years.

I was able to fit the program easily into my lifestyle. Because the workout only took half an hour to complete, I could do it during my lunch hour. The training was challenging but not beyond my capabilities. In addition,

I found the diet plan excellent. The food I was required to eat was very similar to what I usually ate. With the meals spread out into many smaller portions during the day, I found I was not always hungry, and was able to adhere to the plan. I found the recipes to be very tasty and I have continued to use many of them in my current eating patterns.

I wanted to lose some additional weight after the program was completed. To do this, I hired a personal trainer and continued with the exercise/diet plan. After 10 weeks of training and following the diet, my clothes were really loose. I had achieved the weight I had set as a goal. The amount of fat I had lost was around 14 kg and I had gained 3 kg of muscle. In order for my clothes to fit properly, I had them altered. Although I had not been terribly overweight, my blood pressure was higher (135/85 was common) than it was in my later twenties (117/75). After I lost the weight, my blood pressure went back to the value it used to be.

I am continuing to train regularly and my strength is steadily increasing. Strength training is not time-consuming to do, since only one set of each exercise is done to success. It is very effective in increasing strength. As a result of using interval training for the cardiovascular part of the workout, and then moving quickly through the weight-training section, my cardiovascular fitness has improved, and my heart rate has lowered.

JANELLE ZETTEL

AFTER MANY YEARS of hundreds of fitness classes, I was frustrated that I was unable to lose the extra weight I had gained over time. I considered myself self-motivated, and when I met with a personal trainer I warned her that I might be a special challenge. Surely there must be some reason, out of my control, for the persistent excess weight.

Many times I had read the signs in the gym proclaiming the success of a six-week fat-loss program. I dismissed it as an unnecessary expense, but every time the signs went up, my interest was piqued once more.

My son's wedding in June inspired me to take action. I wanted to make him proud and to look the best I could. Most of all I wanted to feel good about myself again. Six weeks before the big day, I began the fat-loss program. It was gruelling. Three times a week I met with the personal trainer and she put me through an intensive resistance-training program. Along with that, I followed a simple, healthy food program, which to this day I still use as a guideline. Imagine how pleased I was to walk down the aisle in a beautiful dress two sizes smaller than I had been six weeks earlier!

This was only the beginning of my transformation. I felt good about my accomplishments, but they were just the catalyst for even greater strides in my battle against overweight. For the entire summer and fall, my personal trainer and I worked toward a healthy goal. Week by week I became stronger, fitter, leaner, and more confident. Even my posture improved, or was I just strutting?

My closet was bare. All of my clothes were much too big and I had given most of them away. All I had left were clothes I had worn 10 years ago that once again fit. When I looked in the mirror now, I saw the woman I once was. My husband couldn't complain when I had to go on a much-needed shopping excursion.

I still work out three or four days a week, and weight training is an important part of my program along with aerobics, sometimes even the occasional fitness class. Of course there will always be new goals and new challenges. I'm not finished with me yet. That's what personal growth is all about.

DALE MARTIN

SOMETIME DURING MARCH 1999 I returned home from a three-week holiday in Florida. I was shocked to find that I tipped the scales at 250 pounds. This was definitely much too heavy for my 5-feet-10-inches frame. A day or two later I attended a company function. An associate whom I hadn't seen in a long time asked me if I'd hit 300 pounds. That was the final straw. His comment was the catalyst needed to trigger a decision I'd been putting off for years. The next day I started a serious diet and approximately a month later I joined a fitness club.

There are two things I understand about myself: (1) When it comes to exercising, I am a procrastinator; (2) When I have a commitment, I always keep it. Knowing this, I committed myself to 20 personal training sessions. I've completed those plus many more. The decision to work with a personal trainer has been a turning point in my life, health, and attitude. I was 235 pounds when I joined the club. By November 1999, my weight had dropped to 212, and I lost 13.75 inches. My blood pressure, which was at the high end of normal, is now almost perfect.

As part of the training I've received, my energy level is up tenfold, my stress level is down, my thinking is sharper, my health has improved, and my self-esteem is at an all-time high. However, all of this conditioning has created one problem — I'm a 59-year-old male, and I can't find anyone my age "young enough" to come out and play with me!

DAVID CRANE

WHEN I JOINED GoodLife, I had no idea how much I weighed but I know it was over 350 (scale maximum), probably somewhere around 400 pounds. My waistline at that time was 50 inches. After a year of hard work, I now weigh 310 pounds and my waist is 38 to 40.

My personal assessment is that I lost 100 pounds of fat, but I put on 25 to 35 pounds of muscle and lost 10 inches off my waist. This was how I kept my New Year's resolution I made to myself.

MARY PRICE

ALL MY LIFE the thought of exercising has sent me running in the other direction. For 48 years I have been a couch potato. I was always the one saying, "You go, I'll stay home and make a great meal for you." As a result, my weight kept going up and I developed extremely high blood pressure and high cholesterol. The only thing that was going down was my self-esteem. As I got older, I knew I had to do something, but I had trained my mind to think it was impossible for me to change. I hated exercising — period.

Then I got a job cleaning a fitness club. As I looked around, I saw people like me, young and old, trying to do their best on their own levels. When I learned about the Fat Loss Program, I decided to join. At first I was scared, but each time I went, I found myself feeling better and better not only about what I looked like but also about who I am.

Now, my weight has gone down, but even better I feel healthy. My doctor couldn't believe my blood pressure. I have energy I never thought I was capable of and when I look in the mirror, I'm no longer shocked by what I see. I'm finished the program now but I am definitely going to continue. One of the best things that has come out of this is that I now love to exercise. I even love the "burn." I love the way it makes me feel about myself as a person. I no longer feel like I can't accomplish anything physical. Now when I fill out those questionnaires in doctors' offices, I can check off the "active" square.

CHAPTER FIVE

A GOOD
RECOVERY

Sometimes life deals us a tough hand. Often books on fitness focus on people who are "normally healthy" and don't take into account that there will be periods in our lives when we will not be altogether healthy, or that some of us may be faced with some kind of chronic health condition or traumatic event. Can fitness play a role in recovery from accidents and illness? Can it help people who have a chronic condition achieve a higher quality of life? My answer to that is a resounding Yes. I know this from my own experience and from the experiences of GoodLife members who have used fitness to aid in their recoveries or to help them cope with health conditions.

My Motorcycle Accident

IN CHAPTER ONE I talked a bit about the serious motorcycle accident I had when I was 19. The accident was life-changing for me, for it was that event that brought me to the career of helping people pursue fitness. I was going too fast, as is usual for almost anyone who rides a motorcycle. A car signalled left, but turned right . . . whack! I didn't want to go through the car's windshield, so I held on as hard as I could to the bike's handlebars. As a result I flipped up and over, my heels hit the roof of the car, I landed on the grass, and the motorcycle landed on me. With a superhuman burst of adrenalin-pumped strength, I threw the 400-pound motorcycle off me to about four feet away. Then I couldn't move — not my head, my fingers, my legs — nothing. Things were going in slow motion in my head, and pain shot through me.

When an ambulance arrived, the paramedics asked me if I could move. I remember thinking, "This is serious." As the sensation gradually came back into my body and I could begin to move my neck and arms, the pain became intense. My whole body was wracked with it. They put me on a spinal board and took me to the hospital. Four doctors had to pull my shoulders back into alignment. There were a lot of torn cartilages, ligaments, and tendons, and my right shoulder was sitting four inches lower than my left. This began my introduction to the world of serious injuries.

Not that I had been injury-free — in my 20 short years I had managed to break feet, arms, legs, fingers, wrist, jaw, ribs, and nose. These breaks were the results of various athletic injuries, stupid injuries, "being where you shouldn't be" injuries, risk-oriented injuries. But the motorcycle accident was really bad, because it involved multiple injuries. I spent a long time in bed convalescing. Then I was introduced to the athletic injuries clinic at the University of Western Ontario. Most other people there were getting treated for various types of athletic injuries. As I learned to use ice, and was taken through all kinds of exercising and stretching aimed at helping me recover, I spent a lot of time talking to other patients and their therapists.

I became interested in how the healing process works. How do you get better after an injury? What drives you to recover and become strong again? For every joint in the body the healing process is different, but general practices do apply: rest, care, stretching, and the overload principle of exercise, "making it stronger faster." You have to apply yourself constantly. The sooner you can make yourself do a movement, the

> *The best time to stretch is after your fitness routine or a hot shower, both of which bring blood to the surface of your muscles. Regular stretching will help prevent injury and make your whole body more elastic.*

better it is in terms of your recovery.

I asked myself, "Why does one person get better faster than another?" Is one stretch better than another stretch? How much depends on the head, on what you're thinking? How much depends on the body? I began to realize that a crucial component of recovery is attitude. When you've always taken your strength and health for granted, you get a major wake-up call when you're seriously injured. Looking back on that time, I can now say that my recovery actually made my body better. It forced me to think everything out. It made me learn how every muscle group worked. It also made me see how hard some people will work when they lose something, while other people just seem to give up and become apathetic.

The motorcycle accident created the life I have today. At the time, as I've mentioned, I was going to go to the business school at the university. I might even have become a banker. But my accident was the catalyst that started me thinking that there is something viable in getting the body to be the best it can be. My goal, to recover my physical strength and to emerge mentally stronger, ultimately led to a career.

When I looked at fitness clubs at the time, what they all had in common was that they did sales. They sold memberships and used all kinds of enticements to get people to buy. None of them really understood fitness. And the people who did understand fitness, the kinesiologists and exercise physiologists at the university, didn't know how to sell people on fitness. When I say sell, I mean they didn't know how to encourage them, motivate them, make them want to participate, make people buy into the fact that they're wonderful and they can do it. I became totally enraptured by the question of how to make people be the best they can be — to help them play a better squash game; to make them stand straighter, get stronger, go faster; to train their hearts and lungs; to help them gain maximum flexibility.

Later, that following autumn, I began rowing. Rowing is a continuous, rhythmic action. It gets under your skin and feels really good, but it's hard work. To do it, you have to be very fit. You have to be strong both muscularly and psychologically. You need good flexibility, phenomenal muscular endurance, and a great heart and lungs. Because of all these different aspects, you have to learn what parts of the body to focus on training during which part of the year, and then focus on training other parts later. You have to learn about training cycles. You have to learn how to go faster, as an individual and as a team, without getting injured. An athlete always operates on that fine edge between exhaustion and exhilaration. Many people go through life like that. They're almost exhausted and they're almost at the peak of their power. For general fitness, you don't have to be that close to the edge.

It was the motorcycle accident and my subsequent experiences as a competitive athlete that led me to the business I am in now. The recovery from the accident, and my status as a high-level athlete who had won five Canadian rowing championships, gave me credibility and also helped me understand something very crucial — what it's like to be on the edge of both very good and exhausted. From that I learned that fitness can indeed be used to push us to recovery from injuries and accidents.

An Injury Can
Be an Opportunity

OFTEN WHEN PEOPLE have an automobile accident or some other
kind of serious accident, it forces them to slow down and
focus on their bodies. All of a sudden they become in
tune with a body they've been ignoring or taking for
granted all those years. Some become resentful that their
body couldn't hold up against two tons of steel. Some
people think the injuries are just going to heal by themselves. That doesn't happen. If there's a major injury, you
need good rehabilitation. As they go through the rehabilitation process, many people begin to think, "Hey, this is
pretty miraculous what I have here — my body's capacity
to heal, its capacity to function — and I'm going to get
that back, or at least get back the best quality of life I
can."

Many people who give it a shot are really amazed at
how fast their body can recover, and they're surprised by
how fast their mental outlook gets involved in the
process. They experience, often for the first time, the
pleasure of doing something really physical. For some
people, the experience of doing rehabilitation exercises
for half an hour every day leads them to establish a lifelong habit of fitness. I've known many people for whom
an injury ended up making their life better. Think of an

injury as an opportunity to discover more about yourself. It's a chance to think of alternatives, to try something different, and to get yourself out of the mindset you were in.

Anybody who does anything active runs the risk of injury. With our increased longevity, almost all of us will have some kind of injury sometime. If you're actively involved in fitness or just active, period, there is a chance you could be injured. But if you don't do anything active, you also risk injury, because you've become weak and susceptible. Back problems, for example, are epidemic in this society. Eighty to 90 percent of back problems are caused by weak muscles. Injuries happen when muscles get weak. If you work on your back, on getting your heart stronger, and on strengthening your shoulders and knees, you'll be able to prevent many nasty, weakness-induced injuries from happening.

I think that doctors always underestimate a person's recovery capabilities. Doctors don't feel comfortable telling you that you can do x; if you don't manage to do it, maybe they could get sued. Doctors can't predict whether you will have the wherewithal to get in there and do the rehab exercises. Doctors are in charge of disease — a state in which the body is not at ease. When they are treating a condition or an injury, doctors have to make the best clinical guesses, based on what has worked in the past and the current state of knowledge about the injury or condition. But for an injury, and for many other conditions, doctors cannot categorically predict the course of recovery. So they will tend to be conservative in their guesses, because they don't want to raise what they think may be false expectations.

A lot of people think they are owed a healthy body, or perfect healing from an injury, especially if the injury was not their fault. For example, if the car that hit yours went through a red light, or your injury at work happened because of inadequate safety mechanisms, you might get absorbed in anger and resentment, and have a sense of entitlement about recovery. The concept of entitlement robs you of your freedom, because you are laying your happiness in someone else's lap. You think you can't be happy unless you get x dollars in compensation or x amount of care. What you have to realize is that happiness is a personal choice about taking control of your own life, and that your recovery is, within the limits of the injury, in your hands.

Many people ask me about injuries in fitness clubs. Overall, fitness clubs have a very low rate of injuries. You can get an injury from overtraining, which tends to happen to athletes. You can get an injury from failing to do something right. Most clubs have standardized equipment that is simple to use and qualified people to show you how. The equipment, if it is good, is designed to do it right. When people get injured in fitness clubs, it's because they're not paying attention to how the equipment works and not doing what they've been told about using it correctly. You don't floor the gas pedal in a car until you have first learned to drive. Some people think they just "know" what to do with the exercises and the equipment. But in this day and age, exercise is a learned skill. You're not born knowing it. When people follow the right procedures and get the right guidance, injuries in fitness clubs are few and far between.

Fitness and Chronic Conditions

LET'S SAY YOU have a shoulder that always hurts. You need to do two things. One is to exercise your whole body so that it reduces the stress on that particular shoulder and what it has to do. The second is to exercise the shoulder so that everything you give it becomes a bit easier. Your body always fails at its weakest link. Your job is to make your weakest link as strong as it can be.

For many of us, our weakest link takes the form of some kind of chronic condition: arthritis, diabetes, chronic fatigue syndrome, heart disease, asthma. A chronic condition is different from an injury. With an injury, you hope for recovery. This can keep you motivated in your exercise rehabilitation. But with a chronic condition, there is no "recovery." There is no pot of gold at the end of the rainbow. There is only "the problem." You can decide whether this can be a good problem. The first thing that often happens when you get diagnosed with a chronic disease is denial. The second phase is self-pity: "Why me?" The third phase is the choice between giving in or fighting.

When I was 32 and I was diagnosed with rheumatoid arthritis, my entire body was filled with pain. My hands and feet wouldn't work. I could barely move. And all this had hit me out of the blue, the day after I had won a rowing championship. Overnight I went from racing in a high-level competition to being an invalid. I thought at first that I had an athletics-induced arthritis. I thought I had brought it on myself by pushing the limits. It never occurred to me that it could be rheumatoid arthritis, even though it runs in my family. The doctors didn't know, either. Nobody thought that I, this fit guy, might have a condition like rheumatoid arthritis.

When the diagnosis was confirmed, the doctors told me not to exercise. I obeyed them for a few weeks, but found I was just getting weaker. In my usual headstrong manner, I decided to go ahead and exercise, just as I had always told everyone else to do. When I got back onto a stationary bicycle, I had to have someone help me turn the wheels. After about six weeks, I could turn the wheels myself. Then I had to have help with the weights, and when I did the strength training everything hurt. But gradually I began to notice an improvement.

With any chronic illness, you need to figure out how to be as strong as you can be, all over. I knew this from my background in exercise physiology. If you can put up with the pain from the exercise, the result is that you'll feel better later. At first I would have arthritis attacks every three months that lasted four to six weeks. Then the attack frequency went to every four months, then every six months, and now it's every couple of years. Not only have the attacks decreased but if I keep building up my strength, it serves me well when I do get an attack. The same endorphins that make the average, healthy person feel good during exercise will help you to feel better when you use exercise to help you manage a chronic illness.

When I was 36 I decided to get into downhill skiing. Because of the arthritis, I couldn't use my shoulders to get up out of the snow. I couldn't hold onto the poles or push on them. When I fell, I would get up by collecting my legs under me and rolling over so that I was lying on my back. Then I would cross my arms on my chest and use my thigh muscles to raise myself up. There was no way I was going to allow arthritis to keep me from skiing. And there are people who ski with only one limb, or without any legs at all, or even blind. Now that's courage!

The older you get, the more likely it is that you will have a chronic condition to deal with. As we age, we need to learn how to deal with these conditions. I consider that my arthritis made my business successful. It made me a happier, more caring person. It made me not take things for granted. When you can't even open a car door for yourself and you have to wait for people to do things for you, you begin to understand some of the problems that other people may have. If you have a chronic condition and you improve the quality of your life by managing it well, your sense of the value of life increases. Even though I may be strong enough today to go outside and smell the flowers or see the stars, I wake up every morning knowing that I might not be able to do so that day. Having arthritis has made me highly empathetic. When someone comes into a GoodLife club and says, "I've never been able to work out," or "I was always laughed at in high school," or "I'm too old and out of shape and I don't feel well," I know what that person is feeling.

Many chronic conditions, such as diabetes, arthritis, or chronic fatigue, are insidious because you can't see them. But these conditions can be turned around to be life-enhancing if you choose how you're going to react to them. Maybe their onset shocks you into taking care of yourself. Taking care, taking control, doing something all give you good hope. In the fitness industry, more and more we find we are working with people who have chronic conditions. The baby-boomer generation forms a large part of fitness clubs' clientele and, as the boomers grow older, they will be confronting their mortality and the physical conditions that go with aging. Increasingly, fitness clubs are designing programs for older adults, aimed at enhancing quality of life and achieving a good level of fitness for each person as an individual, no matter what conditions he or she may be battling.

"Good hope" is taking what is dealt to you and turning it around. It's deciding that you can make the best of what is happening in your life. You could decide just as easily to make things worse. There are people who do incredible things despite great odds. If you're even trying to improve your health and fitness, congratulate yourself and feel good, because many people are not even trying.

> *In everyday living one of the most important things to pay attention to is what happens when you're lifting — groceries, construction materials, laundry — whatever requires you to use strength when you lift. Remember to keep both your chin and your eyes up, because this keeps your spine straight. Bend from your knees. Always be conscious of your centre of gravity, which is located two to three inches below your belly button. Keeping your spine straight and bending from the knees keeps you aligned with your centre of gravity and eases strain on your back.*

If you have a chronic condition, "doing fitness" is not going to cure you, but you will increase your quality of life, minimize the impact of the condition, and maximize your opportunities for health and well-being. Most people don't even know I have rheumatoid arthritis. On average, I'm stronger than most men my age (45), and I always want to have that edge.

Fitness helped these people recover from major challenges:

DONALDA GARLAND

I WISH TO tell you how fitness has changed my life for the better. The story I have to share starts out tragically but ends on a note of triumph. I am a survivor of a violent crime and, despite reconstructive surgery, I was left disabled with crippling pain. This tragedy left me not only physically broken but the person I was inside disappeared. I was always an outgoing and fit person, but this violation caused me to hide away in shame. I turned to food for comfort, and felt safer as my fit and healthy body gained pound after pound.

As time progressed I lost hope that I would ever be able to regain the healthy body I once had. With the love of family and friends, plus the support of doctors and therapists, I was able to regain a sense of self-worth and wholeness. However, the injuries to my body are permanent and there is nothing more that medicine can do for me, except relieve my suffering with drugs. With regret I accepted the fact that I would never be able to go for bike rides or hike a trail with my boys and husband again. The reality of the journey before me often left me feeling full of despair.

However, my life was given a new direction. As a birthday present, my husband bought me a membership to a GoodLife club. I was excited at the thought of exercising again, but at the same time I was fearful that I would injure myself or fail miserably. I couldn't comprehend how I was to travel this road alone.

Fortunately I was not alone. From the first day I arrived at the gym, I have received overwhelming support from the staff. Several of the personal trainers went out of their way to help me get a healthy body. I feel safe at the club, knowing that the trainers are there watching over me with special care. One trainer has often stopped just to talk and encourage me. She listens with care as I share my anxiety over my limitations and self-image. A class instructor takes extra time, one on one, to help me modify the movements my body is unable to perform.

It amazes me how far I have come. I have lost 11 pounds and 17.75 mm of body fat. My strength has improved and my physical pain is more manageable. But more important, I have regained something I thought I had lost forever — the confidence to grow.

Six days a week I awake with a path set before me. Whenever I stumble, the staff are there to help me find my strength to go another mile. I probably will never win a contest or an award for physical excellence, but that is all right. You see, I'm already a winner. I've been given a second boost on the road to a good life.

VICKI HUSBAND

I AM A 46-year-old female who was starting to give up on life. My story begins in 1988 when I was diagnosed with a bone disease called congenital coxa vara, which was causing the deterioration of my hips. In 1988 and 1989 both hips were surgically reconstructed and after numerous months of therapy I returned to work in 1990.

Everything seemed to be going well until November 1993, when I was rushed by ambulance to the hospital with an extremely high fever, pain, and shortness of breath. Days of testing were to no avail and I was transferred to a larger hospital, where a team of doctors tried to figure out what was causing the extreme pain and fever. On numerous occasions my husband was called to return to the hospital because they thought I would not make it through the night. Finally a third-year medical student suggested a bone-marrow biopsy, which led to the discovery of a rare disease called sarcoidosis, which attacks mainly the organs in the body. One of my lungs had already collapsed, my kidneys were beginning to malfunction, and my fevers were still continuing. A new drug was brought in and, along with steroids, it seemed to put me on the road to recovery. Every day I felt a little stronger and finally I was sent home, but still continued with incredible amounts of steroids.

I was in and out of the hospital numerous times, and on one of these occasions they added fibromyalgia to my list of diseases. Fibromyalgia is a muscle disorder that causes great pain and makes doing normal, every-day things almost impossible. When I first went into the hospital I weighed 105 pounds, and then, because of the steroids, I was up to 165 pounds, but was unable to do anything to lose weight.

In 1997 I was struck with lupus and, once again, more steroids. My weight jumped to 206 pounds. Because of the embarrassment I felt due to my weight, I became a hermit and would not go anywhere. In 1998 our best friends' four-year-old daughter, Hannah, was diagnosed with an inoperable brain tumour. This tragedy became my inspiration to do something. I organized three fundraisers to help pay for Hannah's drugs, which were brought in from the United States and not covered by OHIP (the Ontario Health Insurance Plan). Sadly, the drugs were not enough and Hannah passed away, but she had given me the inspiration I needed to make my life somehow better.

I decided to join a GoodLife fitness club. The staff there really cared about me. It was hard work, but they made it fun and exciting. I could not wait to go to the club when I woke up in the morning. It was as if I had a new family. My success is just beginning. I have lost 33 pounds. Just recently, it was discovered that I am having mini-strokes, but no one will keep me away from the club. We have another 30 pounds to go. I truly believe that involving myself with fitness has saved my life.

VIRGINIA ANDREWS

MY ROAD TO better physical well-being started in 1989. At that time I was a frustrated, stressed-out bus driver, and I knew I had to do something to alleviate the problems associated with my job. At the same time I had realized that the peanut-butter sandwiches and potato chips had to go, as I had gained enough weight to make me feel very uncomfortable with myself. My self-image needed realignment. I had also been told by my doctor that my cholesterol count was too high and that I had arthritis in my spine.

With my new-found determination I went on a diet, quit smoking, and started walking to and from work. I also joined a GoodLife fitness club, and in due course I lost the weight I had packed on. My arthritis stopped waking me with grief every morning and my sense of well-being soared. Fortunately, my husband also decided to join me in pursuing exercise.

I really miss my workouts when I'm not able to get out, and I can't imagine life without a fitness program in it. I should also mention that my husband was diagnosed with multiple sclerosis in 1996, and through his own determination he has managed to keep episodes of flare-up to a minimum with his dedication to his regular workout program. Physical fitness is now a regular part of our lives.

DARLENE FLOYD

DECEMBER 1, 1987 — I was driving on Highway 17 on my way to check on a sick friend. Just after the turnoff I was involved in a head-on collision with another car, which almost cost me my life. To this day I still do not remember the accident. What I do remember are the injuries I sustained and the hard road back to recovery. My injuries included 18 broken bones and a compound skull-fracture with a concussion, as well as multiple lacerations and contusions.

Meeting me today, more than 13 years later, it is difficult for anyone to believe that I was involved in such a major car accident. Doctors were amazed at the extent and speed of my recovery. When asked if I belonged to a gym or was involved in regular physical activity, I said yes. The doctors informed me that the reason my body healed so well and so quickly was because of my involvement with using fitness equipment on a regular basis.

JAMES CALDWELL

FROM CHILDHOOD WE are told that life holds many surprises and is full of unpredictable and sometimes life-altering events. Yet we are frequently ill-prepared to face these realities when they show up at our doors. Most of the time we can wing our way through, but once in a while nothing seems to work. So it was in the spring of 1996, at the age of 50, that I faced one of these unexpected visitors.

With a long and painful separation behind me and the reality of losing my nest egg, I took up rollerblading as a means of physically, spiritually, and symbolically getting back on track. The future appeared wide open until one day in May. While I was slaloming down a wooden bridge, the wheels of one skate dropped through a crack as my upper body rotated downhill. Sixteen weeks later, the cast was removed. I was faced with the task of rebuilding a leg and dealing with unsolicited advice about acting my age. Four months of rehab got my ankle working, but my mental edge was gone. My confidence was lacking. My goal of moving forward seemed like a distant dream. Perhaps my critics were right in telling me that a more sedentary life was more appropriate for an "aged warrior."

One visit to a fitness club convinced me to try

another approach. Six weeks later, on my birthday, I stood at the top of the "Elevator Shaft" looking down through the moguls on the ski slope. I had a flashback of standing at the top of the stairs with crutches under my arms, working up the courage to take that first step. It was a new experience on a ski hill to feel the cold chill that comes with fear. Fortunately, another flashback occurred, showing me why I was here in the first place. I remember the feel of the wind stinging my face, and my legs moving in slow motion to their own rhythm, winding through the bumps. Time stood still. Somehow I reached the bottom still on my feet, heart pounding and out of breath, but totally pumped! It was a rush unlike anything previously experienced — and I have never looked back.

More than three years later, I continue to work out regularly and have picked up squash again after 10 years. As far as getting on track again, this life-enhancing experience has opened the door to a new career focus and a relationship I thought was well beyond my reach. And the best part of the story is this: Two years after walking into the club and taking up the challenge, I became the proud and very happy father of a little boy. When asked why I would "start again," I smile and just say, "Because I am blessed and able to do so."

CHAPTER SIX

GOOD BRAINS

E<small>VERYONE KNOWS THAT</small> if you eat good, nutritious food, you will be healthier than if you eat poorly. Everyone knows that if you exercise, your body functions better. Everyone also knows that if you don't get oxygen to your brain, you die. But most of us don't realize that fitness has as much impact on our brainpower as it does on bodies. Improved oxygen flow to the brain improves its capability for thinking, and exercise enables a much more efficient flow of oxygen to all parts of your body, including the brain.

Studies have shown that people who exercise regularly produce more work and score better in tests. They have a more optimistic outlook. They recover faster from anxiety and stress. A direct benefit of exercise is the ability to think more clearly. It's not only because of the increased oxygen to the brain. It's also because when your body is fit and functioning well there is a lack of interference in your normal processes, including your thinking. If your body is functioning well, the brain can focus on what it does best. If your body is consumed with stress, and the body's way of coping with stress is physical movement and you're not giving it physical movement, then you have to rely on the passage of time to take the stress away. And as we know, in a society where stress is more common than a cold, the passage of time is not going to help you recover. If you're

---

What schools should offer:
Every child should have 30 to 40 minutes of daily
physical activity at school. It can be very simple
activitie — running games like tag, or a version of
soccer in which everyone gets a chance with the
ball. Kids love tumbling, gymnastics, running.
Children respond very well to exercise. Our
schools owe it to them to provide for their bodies'
need for physical activity.

---

under stress, you are simply not as efficient. If you reduce the effects of stress with exercise, your brain has a greater capability to deal with the tasks at hand clearly and concisely.

Another way that exercise contributes to brain-power is that it improves the quality of your sleep. When your body is getting adequate physical activity, you will enter REM sleep more quickly and overall have a deeper, more restful sleep. Your body is better able to repair itself naturally during sleep, rather than battling the tiredness that comes from chronic stress. Your body will do the real work of self-renewal. If you sleep better, you think better the next day.

Control
Your Mind

WHEN YOU'RE RUNNING around frantically with too many dead-
lines, flustered, exasperated, and stressed out, you're
not thinking as clearly as you would be if you were
calm, relaxed, and in control. Your heart can operate at
10 or 25 fewer beats per minute if you're in shape than
it can if you're inactive. When your heart is beating at a
lower rate you are more in control, and your thinking is
clearer. It's this mental clarity arising from regular fitness that helps fit people be more productive, make
more money, and lead happier lives. Fit people have the
good life, in every sense of the word. People who exercise regularly seem to be more in control than people
who don't, just as a dog that gets a walk every day is
brighter and more content.

Part of being fit is having the capability to concentrate and be goal-oriented. In the workplace this often
translates into business success. Numerous studies
show that fit people make more money. I remember one
study from when I was in university over 20 years ago
showed that people who made over $60,000 worked out
for six hours a week on average. Because fit people have
a lower stress level and higher productivity, they are likely
to become more accomplished at what they do, and thus

153

> *Companies, if they are smart, see fitness as part of people's jobs. Smart companies encourage their employees to become fit and find ways to encourage fitness activities. Some companies have fitness facilities on site; others subsidize fitness programs at clubs in the community. A smart corporate culture encourages people to take care of their own health. Investing in fitness is not altruism — it's good for the bottom line of productivity and profitability. Smart companies know this.*

make more money.

Enlightened businesses know that fit employees benefit the company. That's why some employers pay for fitness programs for their employees, and some companies even have fitness facilities on site. This is not just a perk. These companies know that any edge they can get in the competitive marketplace is worth it.

But this is true not only of corporate workplaces. Let's take another example: airplanes. Why does a pilot have to be fitter than a bus driver? If anything, flying a plane is a less physical job than driving a bus. The pilot often just guides the airplane using automatic controls. So why do airlines insist that pilots stay fit? Because the pilots need to be able to control stress, stay cool under pressure, and think clearly. You might say that so does a bus driver, and that's true. However, pilots are in the sky. My point is that the higher the mental sophistication needed for a task, the more you need to be fit overall.

Let's take astronauts as an example. An astronaut gets strapped into a capsule and doesn't move more than two or three feet in one direction for days on end. Yet NASA makes sure that its astronauts are excellent physical specimens. Why? Going into space is stressful both physically and mentally, and in that high-risk environment you need your wits about you. Even John Glenn, 72 years old when he last went into space, had the fitness level of a 50-year-old man.

If you are fit, your body is in tune with your environment. You have higher self-esteem and self-awareness. If you feel in control of your body, you will also feel in control of your mind. You will tend to believe that you can do things. A good basic level of fitness allows you to enjoy dancing or playing hockey or walking on the beach, so good fun in fitness activities can lead to good thinking.

Exercise Affects Learning

IT'S WELL KNOWN that active children get higher marks in school. When you look at what is going on in schools in terms of physical education, there are some disheartening trends. The schools that tend to offer the most physical exercise are those that have the greatest responsibility to parents — private schools. When a child goes to a private school, the parents pay for the privilege. Private schools know that physical activity enhances a child's development and learning capability, so they make sure that the children are active.

Most people do not have the luxury of sending their children to private schools. The public school systems have some serious shortcomings when it comes to physical education. Running a physical education program costs more than running a classroom. The gym is bigger, the skills of the teachers have to be oriented to physical education, and the equipment and insurance can be expensive. As a result, public schools have been cutting back because they don't have the teachers with the right skill levels or they don't have the facilities or they don't want to spend the money.

Our schools also still tend to concentrate on developing natural athletes and not paying much attention to the average kid in the gym or on the playing field. What happens in the school system is that the only people who have a chance to get fit are the talented athletes who stand out and who make all the teams. We need to make these programs in schools operate on a level playing field, so that every child will know he or she should exercise and will enjoy the activities. We shouldn't be worrying about whether or not a child makes the team. We should be worrying about whether he or she will have the capability to concentrate on life at hand, to have the self-esteem, energy, and intellect to truly enjoy life and achieve. This is the primary reason that GoodLife Fitness Clubs established the GoodLife Kids Foundation, to help make parents and children aware that fitness is good for them — good for their heads, their hearts, and their souls. We will be encouraging the

High schools should offer regular fitness classes. It would be a simple thing for them to offer strength training at least three times a week — this should be available throughout high school. Too often teenagers give up on phys. ed. classes, so we need another way to encourage young people to focus on fitness.

development of fitness programs that can be accessible to large numbers of children.

It's not hard to get kids to kick a ball around. It's not hard to get them to run around the block. It's not hard to improve their fitness levels. A turning point for me in terms of fitness came in my last year of high school. We went running every day for eight weeks. I remember being the slowest runner at the beginning,

> *If young people don't learn to read or write we consider them under-educated and we say that the schools have not done their job. But it's equally irresponsible to deprive kids of the chance to be healthy. We have a public duty in our education systems to pay attention to fitness.*

and in the top five by the end of the eight weeks. I remember how much better I felt every day. I didn't set out to get into the top five. I actually hated having to run. I thought I was just a big, slow guy. I did play some hockey and high-school football, but sports at that time were not a big focus for me. My father died when I was a child, so, coming from a single-parent household, I had to work at part-time jobs. When I was in high school, I worked 25 to 30 hours a week. But I will never forget the slow, incremental improvements I made as a runner, and how good I felt as my body became more energetic and efficient.

I think the school system needs to wake up, because all the statistics show that we are raising a generation of couch-potato kids. Government is being short-sighted as well in not making school-based fitness a priority, because lack of fitness will be paid for later with increased health problems and greater costs to the health-care system. Preventing children from accessing fitness robs them of being what they could be. They will have more colds and illnesses, and more injuries. They will be at greater risk of heart disease and won't enjoy as many things in life. It's wrong to rob our youth of their natural physical heritage. That's not smart. Unlike a lot of other things in this society, fitness programs for children, in comparison, don't have to take a lot of time or money. It should be public policy that fitness is a priority in our schools. Good bodies lead to good brains. And if we're going to meet the challenges of the twenty-first century, we need as many good brains as we can get.

The effect of fitness on brainpower is unmistakable:

MERRILEE DERK

GOODLIFE HELPED ME instill the "good" into my soul. Since joining GoodLife, I am happier, more productive, and a super-positive person. Also, I have lost 90 pounds, trimmed 10 inches from my waist, 10 inches from my hips, 6 inches from my thighs, and almost 5 inches from my chest. I have now adopted a new philosophy: "If you are not happy, you must change your life." I have changed my life and not only am I happy, but I look good, I feel good, and most important, I am healthy now.

Three years ago I was miserable, at an all-time low in my life. I was approximately a hundred pounds overweight. I tipped the scales at almost 250 pounds. My eating habits were despicable and my self-esteem and confidence had plummeted to the lowest depths of disgrace.

I remember taking the first initiative to try to change my life. I flipped through a phone book searching for a fitness club. As I became involved in workouts, I became very dedicated and felt guilty if I missed a session. The first year I was married to the club. Within a month I quit smoking for good. I developed proper eating habits because I needed better nutrition. Within the first year I shed approximately 80 pounds from my body. Two years after my membership at the club, I completed the Aerobic Instructor Certification course to teach fitness classes.

DONALD D'HAENE

HOW HAS FITNESS changed my life? I've become a poster boy for the life-altering changes fitness has helped me make. It all began on my thirty-eighth birthday. I had always desired to be fit, but although the quest for physical health had been a priority it has also been a lifelong struggle. Every time I'd make some progress in my physical condition, obstacles would appear, such as sickness or back spasms, remnants of a car accident.

I was happy emotionally — great relationship, job, and home — but my poor physical condition hampered my quality of life. Initially with fitness I had modest goals. I realized that expecting immediate change would defeat my purpose. Any improvement would be a victory! The real reward was in discovering a physical and spiritual awakening. And what an empowering experience it has been!

People were amazed at my determination and self-control, and especially the dramatic change in my appearance — from a size 42 to a 34 waist, and a 38-pound loss of body fat in just five months. I don't think I'm a better person, but I think I am a healthier person who has increased his potential in terms of longevity, energy, attitude, and example.

MILES KOMLEN

MY LIFE HAS changed for the better since getting involved with fitness. I have found that it takes courage to make big changes in life. Starting a fitness program was not an easy task for me. Most people know they should probably join a fitness club but are often too intimidated to take the first step. I used to think that I had to lose weight on my own before I could even be seen by other people in a gym. But when I joined the gym, I realized that everyone else there was just trying to do the same thing. It was a question of taking control of my life.

It has made such a huge difference in my personal and professional life. I'm better able to set targets and work toward accomplishing larger goals, both personally and in my job. Let's face it: Life is about getting a little further ahead. You just need the right motivational tools and the stamina to get there. I really am living the good life!

LORI TEEPLE, M.D.

FITNESS HAS NOT only improved my own life but it has also enhanced my ability to save lives as an emergency physician. And it has made me a more effective university professor. Through personal training I have gained the skills to develop and maintain excellent upper-body strength. Having a strong left arm is critically important during intubation (inserting an artificial breathing tube). This strength combined with technique allowed me to save a man's life recently when I performed an extremely difficult intubation. Strength and fitness have increased my success at numerous other emergency procedures as well. I often encourage the resident physicians whom I teach to pursue fitness and build strength to become more adept in their field.

As a physician in a major trauma centre, I "speed walk" up to 12 km per shift, attending to a multitude of patients as well as supervising residents and medical students. It is imperative I maintain top cardiovascular and muscle conditioning to keep up this gruelling pace. Fitness has helped me acquire endurance and the high level of energy required to meet the physical and mental demands of emergency work — especially shift work.

My additional role as an assistant professor makes it essential that I not only keep informed of new developments in medicine but that I continually review the basics to enable me to instruct many students and residents every day. During exercise I have developed a way to study. Twenty to 30 minutes on the treadmill has become useful time for reviewing and refreshing my storehouse of medical knowledge. I have become a curiosity at my fitness club, memorizing and reviewing over a thousand study cards I designed for use during exercise. I even used this study system to help me attain my Board Certification in emergency medicine in January 1999.

CHAPTER SEVEN

GOOD ENOUGH IS GOOD ENOUGH

In MY YEARS as a fitness club owner, I have developed a phrase I use with my staff and with the club members: Good enough is good enough. To me, this is the very essence of a fit and healthy lifestyle — to know when you've reached the point of being "good enough" in terms of your health and well-being. The average age of our members at GoodLife in the year 2000 is 38. We have people who join in their teens and people who come to us in their sixties and seventies, even eighties. The baby-boomer generation makes up a big portion of membership in fitness clubs.

If these same people, especially the young adults and boomers, go to any magazine rack and thumb through the pages of a fitness or lifestyle magazine, they'll find articles telling them how to be perfect. There will be features on how to have the best abdominals or the best biceps, how to run a marathon or do a triathlon. The magazines go on and on about perfection. They give us examples of people who have done incredible things. They create a huge guilt syndrome. If you didn't already feel bad enough that you weren't good at sports in high school and never made any of the teams, every time you pick up one of these magazines and see these "perfect" bodies, you're made to feel inadequate. You're always faced with the fact that the model you see in the photos is 20 years younger than you are, and maybe 20 pounds lighter.

I try to instill in my staff the importance of telling people there is a level of fitness that is good enough. Good enough is the level of fitness you need to have a healthy and rewarding life. To use an analogy, on a highway there is a maximum speed limit, and on some highways a minimum speed limit. There's a maximum speed limit because if you drive a lot faster than that, you risk getting killed or maimed. You have a minimum speed limit because if you drive more slowly than that, you'll also be at risk of an accident because someone may ram into you. In life, the minimum speed limit is not being active. Sooner or later you're going to get injured, or you'll have more illnesses, or people will pass you by because they're more successful and enjoy things more.

The other extreme would be that you drive like a racer through life, constantly over the maximum speed limit. You think that you need to work out six hours a day, and you push and push, because you want that body you saw in a magazine. An athlete always verges on injury in order to be exceptional. It's so competitive in high-level sport that athletes always have to push their limits, and so they risk both injury and mental burnout.

As an average person, you don't need to worry about getting even close to the line. In our clubs we frequently get people asking us, "What if I burn out with exercise?" If you're the type of person who's going to burn out with exercise, it will be from trying to do too much for too long. For most of us, this is not an issue. You're much more likely not to do enough. However, you really only need to do strength exercises two or three times a week, and cardiovascular exercises two or three times a week. For example, using the Fit Fix formula we use at GoodLife, you would do one set of weight/strength exercises per body part to success over eight to 12 repetitions — six to 12 exercises in total. Twenty to 30 minutes in total for strength training three times a week, and a similar time for cardiovascular exercises — that's all you need to do. It seems almost too simple, but it works.

What we try to do with new people in our clubs is find out their needs and goals and when they would like to achieve those goals. Then we establish sensible parameters to help them get there. The key thing is to make the parameters realistic, so that the person can feel it's worthwhile to do the exercises. We break everything down into reasonable goals. When the person reaches the goals, we tell him or her, "That's good. Now all you have to do is keep doing that for the rest of your life." That's why I say, "Good enough is good enough."

Three Stages to Becoming Fit

THERE ARE THREE stages in becoming fit. The first is to stop getting worse. As soon as you stop getting worse, applaud yourself. If you stop putting on weight, that's a victory, even though you may still be overweight. If you stop yourself from losing any further muscle mass and strength, that's a victory. Most people never recognize that. Stage one of "Good enough is good enough" could be that you're 40 pounds overweight and you stop gaining more — that's fantastic!

The second stage is when you begin to work to reverse the damage. You decide how much you want to reverse. Say you are 40 pounds overweight and you decide to take off 20 pounds. When you get to that point, celebrate the victory. Then all you have to do is maintain that level. If you're doing the same weights two or three times a week, you reach your goal, and you keep doing the same thing from year to year, in fitness terms it means you're not getting any older. If you've taken your 20 pounds off and have increased your strength by 100 percent, which almost everyone can do in six weeks, you have reduced your age in terms of your actual fitness age. Chronological age is one thing; actual age is another. If you can do the same things at 40 that you could do at 30 — fitness-wise, you are 30.

The third stage is simply maintenance. That's what I mean by "Good enough is good enough." A small number of the general population, probably less than 2 percent, want to go to their maximum fitness levels. But to be fit you don't have to be at your maximum fitness level. Many people quit fitness programs because they don't realize that just stopping getting worse is a good thing. Or they set goals for themselves that are too aggressive and too fast and then they're not satisfied when they don't achieve them. Or they keep setting further and further goals, when instead they should be saying, "I'm OK." If you fit within the body-fat and strength parameters for your body type, if you can do what you want to do in life, if your stress level is controlled by the fitness activities you do, that is good enough. It should be a non-issue in your life. So when you get to 20 percent body fat, you don't have to push to get to 10 percent. You might just say, "I'm happy with 20 percent because I'm healthy and I feel good." You don't have to become the next perfect bikini figure or the next Mr. Hercules. You have to be who you are.

Staying Motivated

PEOPLE ASK ME about motivation. The best way I know to stay motivated in fitness is to not to chase perfection, but rather to chase "good enough." You realize that you don't have to be perfect. To use another driving analogy, how many people can drive like a professional auto racer? Not very many. If you went by what consumer magazines say, you would think that everyone should have the body of an athlete or movie star, just as if everyone should be able to drive a race car. That's unrealistic. A lot of people would like to be millionaires. But how many are willing to pay the price in terms of the hours and effort needed to actually become one? That's why it's so attractive to dream about winning a lottery or answering the million-dollar question on *Who Wants to Be a Millionaire?* Well, you can't win a lottery that helps your body, but you can win the health game with "Good enough is good enough."

Another big component in motivating yourself is to be happy that you're not deteriorating and becoming decrepit. Even more important, realize that in a very real way you can turn back the calendar on your age. Imagining the months going backward on a calendar or a clock going backward can be a powerful motivator. Most people can get to that stage within three to six

A training routine for good health and fitness should always be done in cycles. Think of it as waves on a beach, coming one after another. Here is the type of cycle I use:

September–November

My strongest focus is on strength training. At the same time I maintain my cardiovascular fitness level.

December–March

During the winter months I tend to be in a holding pattern. I keep my strength and my cardiovascular fitness at roughly the same level. This is great psychologically because you're not always feeling like you have to improve. You go through phases where you can maintain one thing and focus on another rather than trying to do everything at once.

April–August

This is the time I make my cardio workouts harder. A lot of cardio-based activities, such as tennis, hiking, or climbing, can be done outdoors. This makes the summer an excellent time for me to concentrate on cardio while still maintaining my strength.

> *The idea behind training cycles is to focus primarily on one part of your training at a time while maintaining the others. You will become stronger, fitter, and faster if you train in cycles. Remember that your body needs periods of recovery and rest. The periods of rest allow you to focus more intensely when you work harder on the other areas. The older you get, the more rest you will need in between certain activities. Training cycles allow you to adapt your fitness routines to your body's needs, your favourite sports, and your particular lifestyle.*

months. If you make your "real" age 30 in terms of fitness, and you can stay 30 until you're 55, isn't that exciting to contemplate? Every year, the day before my birthday, I test the weights to make sure I'm the same as I was a year ago. On the day of my birthday I test myself on the cardiovascular equipment to check that I'm the same. Then I can say, "Hey, I didn't get older!"

Most people's resting heart rate goes up about one beat per year. So if mine doesn't go up, I'm not getting older. If it goes up only one beat in five years, I'm still staying younger. Let's say you're 50 and your resting heart rate is 65. If the average is 78, that's good. If you exercise and, six months later, your resting heart rate is down to 60, you've just shaved five years off your fitness age. You're not 50 anymore, you're 45 or younger. Resting heart rates can vary, but the improvement is what counts.

Once you have gone through the learning curve of becoming fit — learning how to strength-train and do cardiovascular training — you can just keep doing the same thing. You won't see this in any magazine articles. You don't see articles that say, "Don't change. What you're doing is fine." People might think this could be boring, to keep doing the same thing at the good enough level. Well, so is brushing your teeth, but it's nice to have good teeth. So is washing, but it's nice to smell good and look good. The point is that such a fitness routine is non-stressful and easily maintained. A major benefit is that you give it a small amount of time and reap a huge payback.

Magazine publishers can't sell magazines to you if you think you're OK. Book publishers can't sell self-help books to a person who feels psychologically healthy and is doing fine in life. Sure, we will always encounter problems in life, and it's not necessarily a bad thing to look for advice in books. My point is that you should be wary of those books, magazines, TV shows, and movies that flaunt perfection, because perfection does not exist. Good enough is good enough says "I'm OK." The body is wonderful. It doesn't need perfection. It just needs a level where it can work well and you can feel good.

Good Enough Is Balance

A GOOD LIFE is a state of good balance. What this means is that by making a decision to be fit and then recognizing that good enough is good enough, you can balance everything that is important in your life. Part of the reason that you can achieve this balance is that you have a high level of self-esteem because you've taken control of yourself. Regardless of what anyone else says on the subject, it is widely agreed that part of balance is the ability to cope and to deal with things in a positive manner. Fitness allows you to cope.

When you achieve balance, you establish healthier priorities in your life. When you become fit and your body gets in sync with you, you find that balance begins to extend into other areas of your life. You don't become all-consumed by your work life. You find time for family and friends. You find time for recreation, and for solitude and reflection. In so many people I have seen the decision to pursue fitness carry over into every other aspect of life. It's not important whether you do your fitness routines in the morning, the afternoon, or the evening. Do them when it suits you to do them. When you know what times you are going to devote to your fitness, it will help you establish a time frame for everything else. If you decide to work out before breakfast, then you know what time you're going to wake up. If you decide to work out in the evening, you know what time you need to leave the office or what time dinner will be. Fitness routines will help you establish healthy patterns.

Why do I think fitness should be such a priority in your life? Because your life is a priority. When you decide to be fit, you've decided to take self-control. And self-control leads to balance. When you listen to your body, you listen also to your head, your heart, and your spirit. When you achieve a state of balance, you become aware that there is no mind/body split. You are one whole organism. Everything you do to achieve health and fitness has an effect on your mind, your emotions, and your inner peace.

When you are under stress, as all of us are in this society, with its technological advances and rapid pace of change, your body and spirit deserve the recovery that exercise brings. You deserve to burn off any nega-tivity and anxiety and the effects of overwork and other life challenges. Fitness will help you get through tough times. When life throws you a curveball, if you're healthy and fit you'll find it easier to maintain your equilibrium.

It begins with the body. Think of yourself as a house.

Your fit body is your foundation. An unfit body is an unstable foundation. If your intellect and emotions are the walls, and your foundation is fit, those walls stay up straight and help you hold your treasures inside. If the walls are vulnerable because your foundation is shaky, the house could fall apart. Think of your soul as the roof. To be truly self-actualized, everything below the roof needs to be in good working order. Everything works together to make the dwelling place that is you.

These people always remember — Good enough is good enough:

CAROLYN HYNDMAN

IN AUGUST OF 1999 I made the best decision of my life. I joined a fitness club. I work in the health-care field and I am on my feet a lot. I decided to join because of the swelling in my knees. I had a spare tire and have always had poor eating habits. I've tried dieting and it worked for a while, but with no physical exercise I gained it back. Then I joined the GoodLife Fat Loss program and lost 20 inches. I also joined the Reshape program and lost four more inches. In total I have lost 37 inches and approximately 30 pounds. I try to work out every other day, and I joined a Punch class and another exercise class. I now feel much better about myself and I know I can achieve my goal, because a healthy body is a healthy mind.

PAT POSNO

MAY 1999: THE time was right; my body was ready. This was really important. A second grandchild was born. My body was more fatigued than I wanted it to be. So I made an investment in my health by signing up for some personal training. My goals: I needed an increase in energy levels, an increase in flexibility. I wanted to live longer, enjoy life more, and look trimmer. After eight weight-training sessions and my accompanying cardiovascular work, I felt less tired and walked taller! A slight setback: a broken toe sidelined me for six weeks. Enter Renee — a bouncy, positive, happy, personal trainer. Sometimes I felt nauseated during the exercise and felt an unusual tingling sensation in my arms. We worked together to rectify the situation. Workouts were stopped and reconstructed. We talked about diet and my personal goals. My body adjusted time and time again. No more tingling sensations. The results showed inside and out.

End of July: More inspiration! My son and his wife are expecting twins. Workouts consisted of weight training twice a week. Focus was on proper body position, technique, and breathing. With 18 successful workouts completed, I signed up for 20 more. My hard work is showing and people say I glow. As my resting blood pressure and heart rate decrease, my heart gets stronger and stronger. I can fit my workouts into my work schedule and my private life. This is a new way of life and I love it! I am happier, more focused and grounded.

August: Each week consists of two weight training sessions, two Aqua Works classes, and two Newbody classes. I am having so much fun! More variations by Renee — another fitness assessment that finds my measurements and resting blood pressure are down. Some days are tougher than others, but I always feel much more energetic, both physically and mentally, after my workout.

SALLY ORTBACH

WHEN I DESCENDED the 18 steps into the unknown realm of a fitness club, I saw a sea of black machines, fluorescent lights, white machines, mirrors, and fitness enthusiasts. Unable to imagine myself in this picture, I told the staff that I had never been in a fitness club, had never exercised, hate to sweat, and had no exercise clothes or shoes. Having recently retired, I no longer had the excuse of "no time."

The trainer, Monika, was knowledgeable, tiny, and less than half my age. But she was patient with me and I was surprised that I did not mind the weight machines. Some days I find it really hard to make myself go. Twice I drove and rushed through rather than skip the session. Although I could not trust myself to commit for a whole year, I did sign up for four months. For me it is a big commitment. I do not expect to lose a lot of weight and become beautiful. I want to strengthen my muscles for mobility and do my best to postpone the effects of arthritis, osteoporosis, and other ravages of increasing age.

My adult children are very surprised and proud of me. I have not yet had that "high" feeling from exercise, but I am starting to look forward to my sessions. I am more aware of my muscles and can feel them firming up. When I carried $190 worth of Christmas groceries in from the car, I could actually do it without feeling wiped out. I have increased self-confidence and am now ready to work on healthy eating. When I walk — especially back from the club — instead of mincing steps I take long, loping strides.

BRAD WERSCH

HOW HAS FITNESS changed my life? A number of things come to mind: feeling healthier and more energetic, greater self-confidence, feeling better equipped to deal with the pressures in life, and a stronger relationship with those I love the most.

When my mother went through quadruple-bypass surgery, I began to wonder, "Could this happen to me?" It was at this point that I realized it could happen to anyone. It's been a year and my success has been great. I've gone from 22 percent body fat and 168 pounds to 14 percent body fat and 163 pounds. I lost over six inches on my butt and gained strength and inches in most other parts of my body. I am happy with how my physique has changed over the past year. I believe this has given me the confidence in myself to better deal with day-to-day pressures and uncertainty in life. My self-confidence

185

has grown and I feel more equipped to take on challenging opportunities. I feel healthier, and am able to run farther without getting out of breath. Amazingly, I find I have more time when I make the effort to work out. It somehow stimulates my mind to become more focused and productive.

The most important part of my fitness experience has been that it has allowed me to build a stronger relationship with my wife and children. With my body and mind in better shape, I have the energy and patience to be a better dad and husband. I want my life to be a good life. You should too!

BONNIE WHITTLE

AT AGE 34 I found myself overweight. At 5 feet 6 inches and 185 pounds, I hated shopping for clothes. Everything looked terrible on me. When I finally found an outfit that didn't look too bad, I would buy it in six different colours. I had no energy. I had very poor self-esteem and a low sex drive that started to affect my relationship. I was often asleep on the couch shortly after dinner. This, compounded with a passion for fast food, was leading me down a path of destruction.

I had always fought a weight problem, usually by dieting, resulting in short-term weight loss and a sense of deprivation. In January 1998 my fiancé and I set a date for our wedding. I had only five months to get in shape. I did not want fat wedding photos. Driven by desperation, I called a GoodLife club and made an appointment. I was very impressed from the moment I walked in the door. I was shown the proper techniques on the weight-training machines. Within three weeks I started to feel a difference. This was the first time in my life that I was happy with a start, not desperately waiting for the end results.

When I first started running on the treadmill, I could only run at speed 3.5 for two minutes. I was obsessed with the calorie counter. After a month or so,

I had worked up to speed 5.5 for a full 20 minutes. I started attending fitness classes and found they worked up a good sweat with what seemed like little effort.

I did not like weight training at first, but I persevered. It wasn't too long before I saw serious results, like nicely cut calves and non-flabby arms. Another first to take place in my life was wearing tank tops. Somewhere along the line I lost my passion for fast food. I was now craving healthy foods.

By the time our wedding date rolled around, my dress had been taken in two full sizes. I felt fantastic. I still had some work to do, but no longer felt critical of my body type. I knew at this point I would continue my workouts even though my short-term goal had been achieved.

On New Year's Eve I got to wear very sexy, slim-fitting black pants with a short jacket. Abdominal classes had made it very easy for me to hold my belly flat. I became pregnant in late winter of 1999. I continued working hard through the summer. On holidays I was able to hike and canoe every day. I was in absolute awe about how good I was feeling. On October 20, 1999, I gave birth to a beautiful, healthy baby girl.

I have returned to workouts and am taking it a little slow. I am no longer obsessed with the calorie counter but just enjoy the feeling of an increased heart rate when exercising. I love the way my muscles feel after exercising. I'm looking forward to feeling strong and healthy again. The emphasis is no longer on losing weight, but on actually gaining muscle strength and size.

My life has improved dramatically. I love myself, my life, and my family. My sense of self-esteem has improved and my relationship with my husband has never been better. My husband never once said anything about my old weight, but he's so happy for the way I feel about me now.

I no longer consider fitness to be a "body fix." It's a way of life — the good life.

To be your best,

To be what you could be,

All you have to do is be.

You have to be as strong as you can be.

You need a heart that pumps and is not blocked,

Lungs that inhale and exhale with deep, full breaths,

Legs that stride and run,

Arms that pump,

A straight back,

Good skin, shining eyes.

Make your body your foundation,

The foundation of the good life.

Be your best,

But keep in mind

Always —

Good enough is good enough.

— PATCH

APPENDIX

125 Good Reasons to Exercise

EXERCISE MAKES SENSE, BECAUSE IT

1. increases your self-confidence and your self-esteem
2. improves your digestion
3. helps you sleep better
4. gives you more energy
5. adds a healthy glow to your complexion
6. strengthens your immune system
7. improves your body shape
8. burns up extra calories
9. tones and firms your muscles
10. provides more muscle definition
11. improves circulation and helps lower blood pressure
12. lifts your spirits
13. reduces tension and stress
14. helps you to lose weight and keeps you at your right body weight

15. makes you limber/flexible

16. builds strength

17. improves endurance

18. increases lean muscle tissue in your body

19. improves your appetite for healthy food

20. alleviates menstrual cramps

21. alters and improves muscle chemistry

22. increases your metabolic rate

23. improves coordination and balance

24. improves your posture

25. eases and may eliminate
    back problems and pain

26. alters the way your body uses calories

27. lowers your resting heart rate

28. increases muscle size by increasing
    muscle fibres

29. improves storage of glycogen

30. enables your body to use nutrients
    more efficiently

31. increases the enzymes in the body that burn fat

32. increases the number and size of mitochondria in each muscle cell

33. strengthens your bones

34. increases the concentration of myoglobin, which carries oxygen, in the skeletal muscles

35. enhances oxygen transport throughout the body

36. improves liver function

37. increases the speed of muscle contraction and therefore reaction time

38. enhances feedback through the nervous system

39. strengthens the heart

40. improves blood flow through the body

41. helps alleviate varicose veins

42. increases maximum cardiac output because of an increase in stroke volume

43. increases contractility of the heart's ventricles

44. increases the weight of the heart

45. increases heart size

46. improves contractile function of the whole heart

47. makes calcium transport in the heart and the entire body more efficient

48. helps prevent heart disease

49. increases the level of HDL (high-density lipoprotein)

50. decreases LDL (low-density lipoprotein)

51. decreases cholesterol

52. decreases triglycerides

53. increases total hemoglobin, which carries oxygen in the red blood cells

54. increases the blood's alkaline reserve (buffering capacity)

55. improves the body's ability to remove lactic acid

56. improves the body's ability to decrease heart rate after exercise

57. increases the number of capillaries that are open during exercise as opposed to when at rest

58. improves blood flow to the active muscles at the peak of training

59. enhances the function of the cardiovascular system

60. enhances the function of the cardio-respiratory system

61. improves efficiency in breathing

62. increases respiratory capacity

63. improves ventilation of the alveoli (air sacs in the lungs) for greater oxygen consumption

64. lessens sensitivity to the buildup of CO_2 (carbon dioxide)

65. improves breathing, in that less ventilation is required per litre of O_2 (oxygen) consumption

66. improves bone metabolism

67. decreases the chances of developing osteoporosis

68. improves the development and strength of connective tissue

69. lowers your risk of death from cancer

70. improves resistance to infectious diseases

71. enhances neuromuscular relaxation

72. enables you to relax more quickly and completely

73. alleviates depression

74. improves emotional stability

75. enhances clarity of the mind

76. makes you feel good

77. increases the efficiency of your sweat glands

78. enables you to stay warmer in colder environments

79. helps you respond more effectively to heat, since sweating begins at a lower body temperature

80. improves your body's overall composition

81. increases body density

82. decreases fat tissue more easily

83. helps you make your body more agile

84. increases your positive attitude about yourself and your life

85. increases the level of the hormone norepinephrine, which boosts the spirits

86. stimulates release of hormones that alleviate pain

87. alleviates constipation

88. increases the efficiency with which adrenalin is used, resulting in more energy

89. enables you to meet new friends and develop fulfilling relationships

90. enables you to socialize at the same time that you are getting into shape

91. helps you move past self-imposed limitations

92. gives you a greater appreciation for life because you feel better about yourself

93. enables you to enjoy all types of physical activities more

94. makes your clothes look better on you

95. makes it easier to exercise consistently because you like the way you look and feel and don't want to lose it

96. gives you a greater desire to participate 100 percent in life — to take more risks — as a result of increased confidence and self-esteem

97. improves athletic performance

98. enhances sexual performance

99. improves the whole quality of your life

100. helps you live longer and better, giving you an extra hour of life for every hour of exercise

101. is the greatest tune-up for the body

102. reduces joint discomfort

103. increases your range of motion

104. gives you a feeling of control or mastery over your life and the belief that you can create any reality that you want

105. stimulates and improves concentration

106. brings colour to your cheeks

107. decreases appetite when you work out for 20
minutes to one hour

108. gets your mind off irritations

109. stimulates a feeling of well-being and
accomplishment

110. invigorates the body and mind

111. is a wonderful way to enjoy nature and the
great outdoors

112. increases the body's awareness of itself

113. reduces or prevents boredom

114. increases your awareness of your gait

115. enables you to move from left-brain to right-
brain thinking

116. can change the electrical activity in the
brain from beta to alpha waves

117. increases your ability to solve problems more
easily, and often effortlessly

118. gives you a clearer perspective on ideas,
issues, problems, and challenges

119. releases blockages and limitations in thinking

120. affords you the opportunity to experience your fullest potential

121. reduces illness

122. helps you live longer

123. makes you feel better each and every day

124. makes you feel more alive in your spirit

125. makes people look at you and say, "Wow! You look great!"

WELCOME TO GOODLIFE FITNESS CLUBS

For the latest information on group exercise schedules, club hours and locations, upcoming events, success stories, contests, and corporate information, visit our web site at www.goodlifefitness.com

Contents

DEAR MEMBER:

First, let me offer my congratulations! You've taken the first step towards the Good Life. If you're like most people, you've had to overcome a lot of fears in making this decision. It could be anything from a sense of intimidation about what it would be like to work out inside a fitness club, to having fears such as, "What if it doesn't work?" or "Is it worth the money?" You've no doubt dealt with a whole host of things that you had to overcome so that you could look after yourself and enjoy a high quality of life in the future. So you are indeed to be congratulated!

Second, I would like to thank you for having the trust in us to look after you. I guarantee that we will make sure that you are happy with your decision. This book is just our way of saying we wish you all the best in your journey towards self-fulfillment. We encourage you to read it because you will find in its pages numerous ideas and suggestions that will help you maintain your workouts, sustain your enthusiasm, and reach your goals.

Speaking of goals, we ask you to fill in your goals right here. You can do this on your own or in consultation with GoodLife staff. The idea behind putting down goals in writing is that they become something you can focus on, look forward to, and plan around. So tonight when you're sitting at home trying to decide if you're going to have french fries or chocolate-chip cookies, or whether to go to the club, you have three choices: one — to stay home and have the treats; two — to go to the club and don't have the treats; or three — to go to the club and still have the treats. We encourage you to do one of the last two, both of which involve going to the club. The neat thing about goals is that they drive you in a direction and encourage you to make decisions that support them. **You're halfway there already just by deciding what you want.**

All the best,
Patch

YOUR GOALS

MEMBER NAME: . . . .

DATE I JOINED GOODLIFE: . . . .

LOCATION OF GOODLIFE CLUB: . . . .

MY GOALS FOR HEALTH AND FITNESS
Write down your top five goals and the date by which you want to achieve them:

GOALS	MONTH, YEAR
1.	
2.	
3.	
4.	
5.	

Add any other goals that come to mind that you would like to achieve:

. . . .

. . . .

. . . .

. . . .

GoodLife Fitness Clubs:
A success story to help you!

WHEN I OPENED my first small fitness club in 1979, it was just a 2,000-square-foot facility in London, Ontario. A little over two decades later, we have over 75 clubs, two million square feet of space, 200,000-plus members, and more than 2,500 staff. Our future expansion plans will easily carry the company to over 100 clubs and over 300,000 members. Lots of fun!

CANADIAN ASSOCIATION OF FITNESS PROFESSIONALS

In addition to our clubs, in 1994 our company created an organization to serve the educational needs of our profession. Named the Canadian Association of Fitness Professionals (Can-Fit-Pro), this 10,000-member professional association holds six major conferences annually across Canada. In addition, Can-Fit-Pro offers Canada's leading national certification program. This continually evolving program currently offers the following specialist certifications: Fitness Instructor, Personal Trainer, Program Director, Nutritional and Wellness, Pre and Post Natal Fitness, Older Adult Fitness, Mind/Body Fitness, and Kids and Youth Fitness.

GoodLife Fitness has achieved an impressive array of awards in the past few years:

- 2003 Regional Finalist, Canada's 50 Best Managed Companies.
- 2003 Winner, Consumer Choice Award, Ottawa, for best Health and Fitness Club.
- 2003, 2002, 2001 Winner, Consumer Choice Award, Toronto, for Best Health and Fitness Club.
- Year 2000 Nominee, Entrepreneur of the Year Award, sponsored by Ernst & Young and Global TV.
- 1999 Regional Finalist, Canada's 50 Best Managed Companies.

- 1995 Winner of the Outstanding Business Achievement Award from the Chamber of Commerce.
- 1992 Top Club in Canada by the Club Management Services of the United States, the world's leading consulting company to the fitness industry.

GoodLife's technical expertise is the best in Canada and among the best in the world. The company's retention rate of members is among the highest for multiple club operations in the industry worldwide. GoodLife staff are qualified through national and international certifications in fitness together with physical education, kinesiology, or related science degrees and diplomas.

GoodLife's personal trainers are additionally certified at five different levels: Motivators, Personal Trainers, Master Trainers, Elite Trainers, and Elite Plus Trainers, based on education level and experience.

GoodLife's core values

CARING • TRUST • INTEGRITY • HAPPINESS • PEAK ATTITUDE • PASSION • AND PERSONAL FITNESS.

These are our core values at GoodLife Fitness Clubs. They form our culture and are integrated into all of our member services. Our people exist to serve our members and help each one of them become stronger, healthier, and happier. Our staff, hired with our core values in mind, have the important job of motivating, coaching, and teaching our members. GoodLife emphasizes the selection and training of highly skilled staff, and provides a corporate environment that empowers people as a team and supports excellence at all levels. GoodLife invests in educational opportunities for all staff in the areas of member services, group exercise classes, personal training, sales and marketing, motivational management, and people skills. Our core values are integrated into management meetings, program planning, recruitment, and program delivery. Our staff and management are the soul of our company and, I believe, what set us apart.

Caring sets us apart as a fitness club and as a company to work with. Staff are first encouraged to care for themselves in self-direction, motivation, fitness, and peak attitude. Second, staff are to care for each other as GoodLife team members and to encourage one another to do their best for members and all functions of the club. Third, staff are asked to care for members, to look after their members' needs and interests as if their own.

Caring is the key value and philosophical component of the GoodLife culture. Caring shows which people will be successful in the GoodLife company. It attracts staff who care. It also attracts and keeps the type of members who consider caring to be an important component of their lives and life in general.

In other words, we have decided to be a caring company.

World leader in fitness classes

AEROBIC CLASSES, as these were once called (now known as group exercise), have always been a very important part of GoodLife, but in 1990 I decided that this area should have even greater attention. In 1991 I invited Maureen ("Mo") Hagan, a part-time coordinator and instructor and full-time practising physiotherapist, to come on board full-time to develop and implement our instructor training and certification and to oversee a new department, now known as Fitness Training.

Today that department oversees the operations of all group exercise programs within all the GoodLife clubs and the training and development of 950 group exercise leaders. GoodLife, I believe, offers the greatest combination of quality, safety, variety, and fun classes in the world. The sheer number — over 2,000 classes a week — and choice of classes are astounding. Innovative programs, successful staff training, and incentive programs have helped to attract to GoodLife the best leaders within the Canadian fitness industry, many of whom teach and train fitness professionals nationally and internationally. This achievement was recognized around the world in 1998 when Mo Hagan won the IDEA (International Dance and Exercise Association) International Program Director of the Year award — only the second Canadian ever to have received such an award. Mo was also Bodylife Europe's International Educator of the Year in 1996 and the Canadian Presenters' Choice Award winner in 1997. In addition, a number of GoodLife instructors have their own television fitness shows.

GoodLife created its very own group fitness training and certification program which, over the past 10 years, has been adopted by Canada's largest association of Canadian and international fitness professionals. Can-Fit-Pro, as this association is called, early on laid the foundation for a new Canadian certification known as the Fitness Instructor Specialist. Mo, through her role as Director of Education for Can-Fit-Pro, has helped shape this association to a level where it is now recognized worldwide as the best in the industry.

Caring for future generations: GoodLife Kids Foundation

GOODLIFE CARES ABOUT future generations and is making a significant investment in promoting healthy active lifestyles among children and youth. In 1998, responding to a growing need to support and encourage fitness in children, I recruited a board of directors, and together we articulated a vision and shortly after launched the GoodLife Kids Foundation. A year and a half later, the foundation received charitable status and developed a plan for on-going fundraising to support its initiatives. Those initiatives include educating children about the lifelong health and self-esteem benefits of fitness.

In May 2000, the foundation sponsored the first Kids Power Conference for close to 1,000 grade five students. The delegates experienced sessions on nutrition, fitness, and outdoor activities, and I was the "scared" keynote speaker. I experienced more trepidation facing these 10-year-olds than at any lecture I have given to colleagues around the world! The basis for my motivational talk, called "Climb Any Mountain," was to give these students the thought that to succeed they need the confidence to believe in themselves.

The foundation recently completed a workalong exercise and self-esteem video called Go Kids! Free copies will be distributed to elementary schools and community centres in support of our initiative to get kids more active.

Some time ago I saw an engaging picture of a kitten gazing into a mirror. The reflection in the mirror was of a huge and magnificent lion and the caption underneath read, "Keep up a high sense of self-esteem." This image captures perfectly the essence of our GoodLife Kids Foundation. Children with a good sense of fitness and well-being will have a healthy and positive self-image. As with the kitten, if our youth perceive that they are the best they can be, we will have given our children the confidence of a better future and the feeling that they can positively transform our world.

GoodLife Kids Programs

GOODLIFE HAS CHILDREN'S PROGRAMS and child-minding services in its Loblaws grocery store locations and in most of its other clubs. These programs are designed to be fun, develop self-esteem, and provide the fitness children need. The child-minding rooms are well-equipped, clean, and welcoming. Friendly and caring staff have fun with babies and children alike.

The best way to help your children achieve the Good Life is to introduce them to fitness now for a long, healthy life. It is equally important to be a positive "fit" role model, too — kids copy their parents. We know if your child wants to come to the club you will, too! Get the Good Life together.

"Creating the Good Life . . . now and in future . . . for you, for me, for us all."

The great things GoodLife has to offer you

THERE ARE UNBELIEVABLE opportunities and experiences awaiting you at the GoodLife Fitness Clubs. There are many different forms of strength training, many different types of fitness classes and cardiovascular training, all of which can be quite overwhelming until you get the hang of it. So the key thing is not to be overwhelmed. Just say to yourself, "Look, all I really need to do is some strength and some cardio and I don't need to spend a lot of time — only 20 to 30 minutes three times a week." You don't need to change your entire life's schedule — just a little change will make your life a whole lot better. So it could be that the stuff you learn right off the bat is all you ever do. Or it could be that as time goes by, you will experiment and learn different things. Either way, you win. So that you get the right start, the first thing we offer you is a free, comprehensive orientation program.

Your orientation programs

WHEN YOU FIRST JOIN GoodLife as a new member, you can get started on your program in two different ways. Most members today choose to purchase personal training to ensure that they achieve their desired results through a program tailored just for them. Free orientation sessions are available to all members at scheduled times as well.

PERSONAL TRAINING ORIENTATION

Personal training has proven to give results up to 80 percent better and three times faster than working out on your own. It is the most preferred avenue for any new member joining one of our clubs. Personal trainers are certified Canadian fitness professionals who are dedicated to improving your personal health and well-being. Through teaching, coaching, supervising, and personal support, they motivate and inspire you to your full potential. Personal training is especially effective for individuals getting started for the first time on an exercise program or for those returning after an absence.

Personal training incorporates pre-scheduled workouts, designed to take into account both your fitness and nutritional needs and goals.

As a new member, you will be given a choice of special packages of personal training sessions when you join. These packages are custom fit to individual fitness goals, ensuring success in the first four to six weeks. They also will get you started in the right direction to be able to work out on your own. A fitness assessment and consultation, cardiovascular and stretching orientation, and an individualized program are all included. The real experience comes from the one-hour, incredibly motivating workouts you will receive. It's nothing short of amazing!

GROUP FIT FIX ORIENTATION

The orientation we encourage all new members to try is called the Fit Fix Orientation. You are educated about basic strength-training techniques. We teach you how to use the circuit-strength equipment, how to use your workout card, and the benefits of strength training. You learn how to begin with nine exercises. Those nine key exercises are the ones that give you overall general strength. In half an hour you learn the basics that will allow you to have a successful strength program for life. In conjunction with your strength-training program, you will be given a cardiovascular training program (more about the benefits of these later). Don't miss it!

These orientations at GoodLife are group sessions where your fitness program is designed for you and you are educated on all aspects of your fitness program. This orientation is done in a group of two to six people and is an hour-long appointment. You will have an opportunity to be introduced to and to participate with other new members. It's a good time to make new friends to connect with when you come to the club.

Another benefit of our orientation sessions is that in our program you can take an unlimited amount of orientation sessions. You can take the same session again and again to feel 100 percent comfortable with it, or perhaps if you have skipped your workouts for a couple of months you might want to come back and get a refresher — a do-over, as we say. You don't have to feel intimidated. You can, in essence, start over any time you want. It's casual, it's fun, it's relaxing, and you get to meet other people.

These orientations teach you how to train on the different treadmills, cross-trainers, cross-aerobic machines, recumbent bicycles, stairclimbers, upright bicycles, and perhaps rowers. Our goal is that you know how to train properly to get the best effects in the minimum amount of time. Sounds good, doesn't it? It's part of the Good Life!

GROUP EXERCISE ORIENTATION
All the GoodLife clubs offer Group Exercise orientation and technique classes. These orientations are designed to accommodate all types of members:

• New members, who need to learn about the program and have a fitness program designed for them.

• Current members, who need a refresher on their program.

• Experienced exercisers, so they can learn the specific technique necessary to get the maximum results from their workout.

Remember, the orientations are available to everyone: you

may attend as many as you like and are welcome to join in anytime!

By teaching you the basics of the GoodLife Group Exercise core programming, you know you will have the skills needed for each of our mainstream programs. The instructor can help show you options and is available to go into detail and answer questions you may have. Make sure you sample a class. You will find out that exercising in a group setting is great fun and motivational, leaving you wanting more! The other thing that happens is, you will be pushed to accomplish more than what you could possibly do on your own.

Everyone feels the same in the beginning, a little bit unsure or slightly intimidated by the new surroundings. It won't last for long. As soon as the music fills you with motivation and the instructor cheers you on, you will be on your way. Speak up when the instructor asks, "Is anyone new today?" They are there to help and see that you get the most out of the class.

Group Exercise is a lot of fun and is one of the best ways to get results fast. I would recommend it as part of your balanced exercise program. Every club will provide orientations in each group fitness area that they offer. These may include cycling, rowing, and group aquatics as well as fitness classes. The club's staff will inform you of the schedule for these programs and you can sign up for as many as you like. The fitness boards in each club and Group Exercise schedules will also provide you with additional information. Group Exercise schedules are now available on the GoodLife website for your convenience.

Member ambassadors

WHILE YOU ARE WORKING OUT, you will notice staff associates circulating throughout the club wearing yellow shirts identifying them as a Member Ambassador. These Member Ambassadors are scheduled to be in the workout areas during the busy times to assist you with any questions you may have about your fitness programs or inquiries you may have about other programs available to you.

Our Member Ambassadors are available to assist you with your technique, provide you with a fitness tip, or just be there to smile and say "Hello." I encourage you to use their services to maximize the time you are investing in improving your health and fitness.

Member Ambassadors also provide orientations during pre-scheduled times throughout the week. No sign-up is necessary and you can attend these orientations as often as you like. These orientations are for new members or current members who need a refresher.

That's just a summary of some of the orientations we have in the clubs. Each club is a little bit different depending on what city it's in, what facilities it has, etc. As I mentioned, some clubs have squash or tennis, some clubs also have swimming pools.

As you can see, there is no end to the learning opportunities you can have at GoodLife and no end to the variety that you can experience for yourself. The wonderful thing is that you can feel good about doing the same program and maintaining your great results because "enough is enough," or you can have an endless variety and opportunity of different things to try.

What cardiovascular exercise is and how it helps you
HELPING YOUR LUNGS

Oxygen is the fuel of life. The more efficiently you can take oxygen into your body and expel carbon dioxide, the easier it is to breathe, the easier it is to think, and the easier it is to exercise — the easier it is to get through life in general. It's part of the Good Life. So cardiovascular exercise, simply put, greatly increases the efficiency of your lungs!

Cardiovascular exercise helps your lungs because it increases your efficiency in taking oxygen out of the air, and your efficiency in exhaling Co2 (carbon dioxide) from your lungs. Your lungs extract oxygen out of the air, which is 21 percent oxygen, and take it into your lungs. Your lungs put the oxygen into your blood. Your blood circulates and takes the oxygen to all the organs and cells in your body to use it as fuel the same way fire uses oxygen to fuel the fire.

HELPING YOUR HEART

Your heart's job is to pump the blood that carries the oxygen. Your heart is about the size of your fist. From strength exercise it gets thicker, so it can pump harder per pump, putting through more blood at one time. As you strengthen your heart from cardiovascular exercise, your heart grows in size and volume, too. That means it grows in three ways: the volume of blood it has to pump, the number of times it can pump per minute, and the amount of blood it pumps at one time. If you can pump more blood at one time, your heart is actually able to beat less often while doing the same activities. This means everything is easier. You also have more capability to do anything at a higher level. Our Healthy Heart program is a wonderful way to get your heart in shape and understand it all. That's the Good Life.

UNDERSTANDING YOUR HEART RATE

The average person has a resting heart rate of 76 or 78 beats per minute (by resting heart rate we mean how your heart works when you are not doing anything, just sitting around). It's not uncommon for an Olympic athlete to have a resting heart beat in the low 40s or the mid-30s. If the average person's resting heart rate is 76 and the Olympic athlete's is 36, there is a 40-beat difference. That means the Olympic athlete has 40 more beats' capability. That means they have almost 50 percent more capability for exercise or work than someone else. At rest, they rest

50 percent more — not a bad deal, is it, for just a little exercise!

The maximum heart rate of people in their early 20s is usually about 220. So if the range for the Olympic athlete is between 36 and 200, he or she has a range of 150 beats, where if someone's resting heart rate is 76, his or her range is only 110 beats. So the Olympic athlete can do more exercise, can do more work. Your goal as an average person (in other words, you're not an Olympic athlete) is to get your resting heart rate down 10 or 20 beats so you can do more work, have more fun, and give your heart a rest. Then when you want to go and do something, you have a greater range to go "up" in terms of heartbeats so that everything you want to do is easier than it is for someone who's not in shape. Sound good? It's part of the Good Life.

As you get older your maximum heart rate decreases. One of the benefits of cardiovascular fitness is that the decrease occurs much more slowly, if at all. You might be 50 years old and still have a maximum heart rate of a 35-year-old because you've always stayed in shape — which is why sometimes you'll see people in their 50s, 60s, and 70s beating people much younger. They simply haven't gotten "older." They've maintained their youth. Their physical body is still at a young age even if they have actually gotten older in years. Sounds like the Good Life, doesn't it?

CARDIOVASCULAR EXERCISE AND HEART RATE TRAINING ZONE

If you've ever heard the word *cardiovascular* in terms of exercise, what it means is strengthening your heart and lungs. A lot of things are involved in cardiovascular exercise, but in essence it is really just knowing how hard your heart is working. Two things tell you how hard it's working. One is how hard you're breathing, and the other is what your heart rate is. We teach you how to measure your own heart rate from the pulse in your neck or your wrists. After a couple of times doing this, you'll be a pro.

Then we teach you how to establish a heart rate training zone, which is usually between 50 and 70 percent of your maximum heart rate. Your maximum heart rate, quite simply, is figured out by taking 220 minus your age and 50 to 70 percent of that is the range you want to work in. If you've never worked out before, you will get a cardiovascular program that's actually as low as 30 to 40 percent and you'll quickly work up to 50 percent. Now if you work out at over 70 percent, you're working out at the border range between aerobic and anaerobic. Aerobic means working with oxygen and anaerobic means working without oxygen. The latter is when you're really pushing it. For general fitness you don't need to go over 70 percent. Once you know by measuring your heart rate how hard you are exercising, we want you to be aware of how hard you're breathing. This is called "perceived exertion." After a while you'll know how hard to exercise just from your heart rate (i.e., your perceived exertion).

REWARDS

The combination of maintaining a higher maximum heart rate and having a lower resting heart rate allows the greatest flexibility in your fitness and lifestyle. At the same time, we've talked about how very active exercising burns calories, which is a nice benefit. As well as burning calories and fatty triglycerides, you burn off the chemical reactions to stress that happen in everyday life. Great! The big bonus is that the body rewards exercise by releasing hormones called endorphins, which simply make you feel good — that feel-good feeling you get after playing ball, swimming, or dancing is the body saying thanks, do it again! So there are enormous benefits in cardiovascular training. In summary, you get the Good Life from cardiovascular training because you lower your stress, you burn calories more efficiently, you live longer, feel better, and live easier. That's the Good Life.

What strength training is and how it helps you

YOU SHOULD STRENGTH TRAIN so that you can enjoy the Good Life. Strength allows you to have a life. By that I mean it removes the obstacles, the pain, and anguish that can come from being weak. Strength training stabilizes the joints in your body first and foremost, and protects your skeleton from injuries because it builds up muscles that protect your bones. Strong muscles protect the joints by allowing the muscles to take the weight off them. As an example, when people who have arthritis get stronger and maintain their strength, they cope better with their inflamed joints.

As you get stronger and maintain your strength, everything is so much easier. If it's hard for you to turn a doorknob because it requires, let's say, five pounds of strength, this makes your day longer and harder. But if turning the doorknob is easy because you have a hundred pounds of strength in your hand, you don't even think about it. Well it's the same with everything else. If it's easy to lift up the bag of groceries out of the car because you don't have to worry about a bad back, you're nice and strong, life is so easy. But if you have to think twice about it, if you have to be careful, if you have to reduce the weight of the bag to under 10 pounds or under 20 pounds or under 30 pounds, it compromises your quality of life. If you can carry whatever the bag can hold, everything is so much easier.

Let's look at another example. Let's say you're teaching a child how to ride a bicycle. You can stabilize the bike for him and help him by running along with it. You have the balance and strength to go half a mile, a mile or five miles. It's so much better than not being able to hold the bicycle for someone else because you're too weak.

Think of the benefits of strength training from a very simple point of view. Most people tend to think of strength training as something Olympic athletes or bodybuilders do. But they're at the extreme end of the spectrum. Strength training is something that everyone needs to do just to enjoy an everyday quality of life, just to enjoy all the simple things. It should be easy to carry your brief case or your gym bag or a suitcase and not become exhausted. Yet why do seniors, the elderly, get tired? It's because they get weak. Stay strong and you don't get old. That's also the neat and wonderful thing about strength training. You can do it at any age — you can do it at 10, you can do it at 90. No matter how old you are, independent of fitness level, the body responds positively to strength training and you can double your strength in six weeks to three months.

What happens if you don't strength train? Well, assuming you had some strength to start with, from the time you're 20 onward, you will lose about 5 to 7 pounds of muscle every decade you don't exercise. That means that your metabolism — how much you can eat — decreases about 10 percent per decade. Yet if you only did two months of strength training you'll add 3 pounds of lean muscle mass back on. This is good! That would give you a 7 percent increase in your metabolism. So you can just turn it around. Add on 5 pounds of muscle and your metabolism is back up 10 percent. It's wonderful what strength training can do for you.

Strength training does a number of other things as well: It increases the bone density, it stabilizes your joints, and it helps fine motor co-ordination and gross motor co-ordination. By that we mean it helps holding a pen (fine motor co-ordination) or kicking a ball (gross motor co-ordination).

How do you train for strength training? It's simple. GoodLife Fitness Clubs has the patented Fit Fix formula. The Fit Fix formula entails 6 to 12 exercises in 10 to 20 minutes, two to three times per week. These exercises are done on circuit machines such as Nautilus, Life Equipment, Keiser, Hammer Strength, etc. We have up to six or seven different types of circuit machines depending on the club. In this program you exercise the large muscle groups first, working towards the small muscle groups. Why the large ones first? What happens if you exercise, for example, the biceps of your upper arm first before the chest? If you tire your biceps first — you won't be able to work your chest properly. So you always start with your large muscle group first. The exercises take about 60 seconds on each machine, and a couple of minutes to move to the next machine — it doesn't take long to fit it all in. The nice thing about the machines is that they're simple and if you do them all correctly, as you will learn from the orientations, it's pretty well impossible to get hurt. You simply do 8 to 12 repetitions on 6 to 12 machines and you only need to do one set. You'll get 98 percent of the results from one set as you will from doing multiple sets. If you learn to work to success, which is to exercise as hard as you can, you'll get the same results from doing one set in total as you would from doing multiple sets — and the neat thing is it doesn't take any time. You get the whole thing done in 20 minutes.

We do encourage you to do a five-minute cardiovascular workout on a piece of cardiovascular equipment to warm up before you do your strength training. We do this for two reasons. One, it takes you from whatever mindset you're in and gets you thinking about doing something nice for your body. Two, it gets some of the blood away from the organs in your body to the surface muscles so that they're better able to work because they're nicely warmed up. You can also improve your strength through classes like NewBody or Body Pump or using free-weights. If you would like to do free-weights we encourage you to use a personal trainer to develop the skill levels needed for them.

The Fit Fix is easy to learn after one or two orientations and is a nice way to maintain the Good Life. Another benefit of the Fit Fix program for most people, other than highly trained athletes, is that you actually improve your cardiovascular fitness, too, because you're keeping your heart rate up for up to 20 minutes. Although your heart is working harder when you're actually exercising on the machines than it is before and between the exercises, you are doing what is called interval training. Your heart goes up and down but overall you get good improvement. For most people, a continuous Fit Fix workout is equivalent to running two miles.

The second part we encourage you to do is to improve your flexibility and strength by doing your Fit Fix with two seconds in the positive movement (as you move the weight away from your body) and four seconds as you lower the weight. You're 40 percent stronger as you lower the weight — this is called negative resistance. You take twice as long to lower the weight — so you don't just drop it. This means you actually have to hold it, which allows you to strengthen and stretch the muscles. Doing the weights in a two-second/four-second count also allows you to strengthen your ligaments, which connect your bones, and your tendons, which connect your muscles to your bones. Imagine an elastic band. If you just pull the elastic really fast, it breaks, which is like dropping the weight or throwing the weight up; however, if you pull the elastic slowly, the elastic will stretch twice as far, which is what you're trying to do for your own muscles, tendons, and ligaments. Stretch muscles slowly, exercise them carefully, and they'll last a lot longer and be stronger.

So you can do Fit Fix three times a week in 60 minutes and get fantastic results. You can easily do it for the rest of your life and just maintain those results. Stay young and strong. That's the Good Life.

The Fit Fix concept is used as strength training but it's also used in our Group Exercise program where our classes are a half hour in length, with a warm-up, a cool down, a strength component, and/or a cardiovascular fitness component. This allows you to do just one class and get all your results and work hard in that half-hour. Or if you're one of those people that would like to stay longer, you can put two classes back to back. Most people feel good about getting a good workout in a short period of time. Similarly, we encourage you when you do cardiovascular fitness on the StairMasters, treadmills, cross-trainers, bikes — all the different choices you have — to go for 20 to 30 minutes. You'll get 98 percent of the results in those minutes compared with what you would get in two hours. Plus, you'll be encouraged to come back because it's quick and you'll keep doing it year after year because it doesn't take that much time out of your life. We want you to get the Good Life, not use it up.

What flexibility is and how it helps you

FLEXIBILITY IS ONE of the key ways to stay young and to enjoy the activities you want to do. It's pretty easy to keep your flexibility if you do your strength exercises slowly and carefully. If you do group exercise classes, that also helps your flexibility. If you do your cardiovascular exercises through a whole range of motion, that is another way to help your flexibility. It's a nice thing at the end of your workout to stretch out on the floor for five minutes afterwards, using the stretching as a chance to decompress, relax, rejuvenate, and say, "Hey, I did something really good for me."

Stretching isn't difficult. It should be slow and smooth. Just kind of enjoy it and feel your body. Stretch in the shower, too. Effective stretching that benefits your body is something you get to gradually. You can't do it in one day. You just work a little bit at a time. Don't expect too much and you'll be amazed at how you will stay young and flexible.

Sometimes people have a particular part of the body that is hard for them to stretch or that they don't know how to stretch. Feel free to ask any of our staff, or have a personal trainer give you a special session just to work on the part of your body that needs the extra help. It's pretty normal for people to have different parts of the body be tighter than other parts just because they strain too much in one area or another. There are so many stretches we can help you with that there is no need to feel restricted. Stretching is another way to enjoy the Good Life.

What Group Exercise is and how it helps you

WE'VE BEEN TALKING about the benefits of cardiovascular exercise, strength training, and flexibility. At GoodLife Fitness Clubs, you have the option of working out in your own exercise routine, using a variety of equipment, or you can enjoy the benefits of exercising with a group. You can even do both! The opportunity to do group exercise provides a lot of positive benefits for body, mind, and spirit. The success and fun of group exercise classes depends on that wonderful chemistry we call group energy.

Together Everyone Achieves More (TEAM). In group exercise that is what it's all about. Participating in an exercise program in a group atmosphere with great music and motivating leadership that entertains and inspires you leads to more than just good physical results. Group interaction creates a significant emotional experience and commitment. Thousands of GoodLife members attend group exercise classes for some or any one of these reasons.

Group energy presents itself in many different formats at GoodLife. You might take the group exercise approach to studio fitness classes, aquatic exercise, indoor cycling, and rowing. Specialized programs target specific interests - for example, children, mind/body wellness, martial arts, women, older adults, and new member orientations. All these programs are fun and easy, and we hope you'll join in. You'll be glad you did!

Each GoodLife club has between 20 and 50 classes every week on the club schedules. These classes attract 50 percent of our clubs' members on a regular basis, which far exceeds the industry standard for group participation within a fitness club. At GoodLife we have always been leaps and bounds ahead of the fitness industry in our group programming. We have successfully provided members of all ages and fitness levels with creative and effective class experiences.

While participation in group exercise has declined over the past number of years in clubs throughout the world, participation at GoodLife is stronger than ever. Consistency, reliability, branding, and marketing are key. In 1999 GoodLife introduced pre-designed programming known as Body Training Systems. Since then we have successfully introduced five core programs into the clubs that today, along with our Newbody program, constitute our core menu of Group Exercise programming. Group Exercise at GoodLife is unique, guaranteed by the company's exclusive rights to all six core programs.

Commitment at GoodLife works both ways. The member makes a commitment to a Group Exercise class and looks forward to working out with classmates. These classes are great places to meet new friends! Our instructors are equally committed to the class members. Instructors are given the opportunity to teach the same classes each week for an entire schedule, which is about eight to 12 weeks. This allows instructors to get to know you and how best to keep you, as an individual, motivated. You never hear about members who complain or quit because they have too many friends or because they are having too much fun! Relationships create the energy to succeed, and success creates commitment. Commitment brings about greater success.

GoodLife offers new member orientation classes on a regular basis. When you join one of our clubs, a membership consultant will sign you up for one of these orientation classes. It is important that you attend. GoodLife also offers specialized classes and small group specialty programs such as Women on Weights, Fitness Fore Golf, and CORE Circuit. These will be promoted on either the Group Exercise schedule or fitness boards within the clubs.

We change the schedules to give you a feeling of a fresh start and keep you interested. Group Exercise is more than just exercising in a group — it's about being part of something special and having a sense of belonging. When you feel that you belong, you feel energized and good about yourself and others. That inspires you to be the best you can be. Research shows that if you work out with a buddy or significant other in your life, your commitment is greater by 50 percent. You will find a whole bunch of people to exercise with in our classes and this will keep you coming back for more! Admit it, you would rather work out in a group the majority of the time. Most of our membership agrees with you!

WHEN YOU ATTEND A CLASS FOR THE VERY FIRST TIME:

- Introduce yourself to the instructor and let him/her know you are new to the class. Inform your instructor of any precautions or special limitations that you might have as a new participant to that particular class. Don't be shy!
- Wear comfortable clothes that allow freedom of movement and supportive footwear (a workout shoe or cross trainer is recommended).
- Pace yourself and use perceived exertion (how you are feeling) as your guide for intensity. You should feel that the exercise is somewhat hard but manageable, or monitor your heart rate and keep it within your desired training zone (50–70 percent of your maximum heart rate).
- Bring a friend or buddy — it's more fun and the experience is greater when you can share it with someone.
- Start with the simplest version of the exercise to allow your mind and body to get used to it and learn the skill.
- Focus your attention on correct alignment and form and remember that it is not how many you do but how you do each one that counts. Think quality, not quantity. Begin with the options given by the instructor. Consider the first class in any program as a technique class. Keep it simple and succeed.
- First, have fun and decide to be happy.
- Set a specific goal for yourself for each class and monitor your success. Setting up a workout card or workout journal will help you do this monitoring. At the same time, make appointments in

writing with yourself at the beginning of each week and keep them. It is like paying yourself — the payment is your health.

• Try a variety of classes and aim for three per week: one cardiovascular conditioning class such as Newbody or BodyCombat; one strength training class (BodyPump); and one mind/body class (BodyFlow or a stretching class). Change your program somewhat every six weeks at least to keep it motivating and results-oriented.

• Begin with a Group Exercise class and be sure not to miss out on any of our "release classes" — another great way to get introduced into Group Exercise.

• Respect warm-up and cool-down time to guard against injury.

• Provide the instructor/club with your feedback so we can continue to provide you with the best service.

What personal training is and how it helps you

EVERYBODY'S DOING IT. You should be doing it. Why should just the rich people get the best? We all deserve to look after ourselves. Personal training is the fastest-growing segment of the fitness industry. This trend is expected to continue, as personal trainers offer a variety of services and motivation that go far beyond a general exercise program. They educate, motivate, coach, advise, supervise, and support you every step of the way. The personal training profession will be one of the most sought after career choices of the 21st century.

People maintain and spend money on their cars, houses, lawns, pets, etc. In fact, the average person spends over $600 on just getting his or her hair cut and styled each year. So doesn't it just make sense to use professionals to help you invest in a healthy body and healthy mind? Your attitude should be nothing but the best for your body. It's your most important asset. It requires investment like anything else of value. Your body is more important than your house, car, or clothes.

At GoodLife we really do believe that we can be most things for most people. There is so much to choose from, GoodLife offers you an excellent range of specialized services to make your personal training experience complete and to ensure you reach your goals. Inquire about the following personal training specialty programs:

- The Summer Sizzler Body Makeover Program is set up so that you train once a week with a personal trainer and receive education on different topics such as nutrition and exercise. A great way to get yourself into summertime shape in just six short weeks! Expect an unparalleled workout with phenomenal results.

- The Winter Waister Body Makeover Program is another fat loss option for busy people to train in the winter. This easy to manage program sees great results and you only need to show up with your trainer once a week!

- Group Training is for two to six people and is adaptable to any type of training you want. It's a lot of fun and training as a group brings down the cost.

- The Fit Fore Golf Program will get you in shape for your golf season with exercises and stretches specifically designed to improve your golf game. Get a head start on the season and with greater endurance and flexibility you will excel!

- The First Step Learn to Run Clinic is for new or beginner runners. We will help you work up to a 5 km run supported by two trainer-led group runs each week. In addition, you will receive a running information manual, training schedules, log book, fun, and lots of camaraderie!

• W.O.W. equals Women on Weights. This fun, 60-minute, group specialty training approach to working out uses a variety of resistance equipment such as bands, dumbbells, and barbells or the club's weight circuit format. This program teaches how to safely and effectively train with weights and provides tips on nutrition, flexibility, exercise, posture training, and more!

• Core or Core Circuit Training Program, as it is called, is a group training program that helps you shape up your waistline and fire up your center of power at the same time. You will learn how to improve your posture for both performance activities of daily living and strengthen muscles that you need for a healthy, pain-free back.

• The Body Results Opportunity Session utilizes a unique tool called the Body Composition scale. In just a few minutes our members can have a full Body Composition Profile. It's quick, user friendly, non-invasive, and accurate! You'll receive a full educational booklet customized with your individual body composition data. This five-page colour-illustrated manual includes:
- Total Body Weight
- % Body Fat
- % Lean Mass
- Blood Pressure
- Heart Rate
- Total % Body Water
- Total Daily Caloric Expenditure
- Disease Propensities and Related Risks

Find out if you're healthy Inside and Out!

• BodyFit60. Mike McLeod and Jack Hewitt are two of our personal trainers at GoodLife and the creators of a highly effective fitness program called BodyFit60, a series of detailed resistance training/fitness programs that have been designed to stretch both your physical and mental boundaries. By applying BodyFit60's time-tested training principles and implementing exciting training techniqes, success with the exercise training series is ensured. In just 60 days of one-on-one training, you can achieve fitness success and learn to live a lifetime of health and happiness. Included in every BodyFit60 program is a meal planning guide that provides a variety of recipe suggestions to help you plan your week and understand the importance of balancing both exercise and nutrition. Included also is a comprehensive assessment of all nutrients, vitamins, and minerals, all explained in easy to understand terms. Learn how to calculate your individual daily caloric intake and boost your metabolism with the BodyFit60 fitness series. The workout programs combined with the nutrition information should enable you to combine all the benefits of a healthy, balanced lifestyle. To find out more about the program, visit www.bodyfit60.com.

TOP REASONS FOR PERSONAL TRAINING

1. Studies prove you achieve your results three times faster than exercising on your own.

2. You receive individualized programming for your body type and for your specific needs and goals.

3. You experience unparalleled motivation and increased self-esteem.

4. You can maximize your time with pre-planned workouts.

5. You receive "cutting edge" information in training and nutrition.

6. You learn safety and injury prevention.

7. You will advance past plateaus.

8. You receive professional guidance and expertise.

9. You will be exposed to variety in types of training to keep

you motivated and help your personal growth.

10. There will be a progression of routines to keep your workouts fresh and interesting, designed for you and your lifestyle.

11. You always have someone interested and concerned about your fitness and health.

Here are some questions people often ask about personal training:

Why do I need a personal trainer? Can't I just do all the exercises on my own?
The greatest temptation in all exercise programs is to quit after the first eight weeks, which is why at GoodLife you can restart your orientations at any time you want. It is easy to quit on a program, for we all know how so many other things can seem to get in the way. Through no fault of your own, this has probably happened to you on a number of occasions. Personal trainers know the pitfalls and how to help you avoid them. Their motivation and direction will help keep you on track and help you achieve the results you want. They're your personal "do it" coach. They will inspire you to be your best and feel your best. They are with you every step of the way to make sure you are successful.

Isn't personal training something only movie stars and athletes do?
Personal training is for everyone. It's about becoming the best you can be, regardless of your shape, size, gender, age, or ability. Personal training programs and pricing can be designed to fit everyone's needs. Personal training can be one-on-one or in a group. You will be surprised at how accessible and affordable personal training is for you.

Does it take a lot of time to have a personal trainer?
No, your workouts are normally a half-hour to one hour. I use a personal trainer now for my 20-minute Fit Fix workouts, even

though I've been doing them for over 20 years, and I've noticed a 40 percent increase in my strength!

Will a personal trainer really make a difference?
Yes! Studies have clearly shown that people who work with a personal trainer are 80 percent more likely to achieve the results they want.

GoodLife has the top Personal Training department in Canada with over 700 certified personal trainers to service any client's needs. Here are the top reasons why we believe we are second to none.

1. Every GoodLife club has a personal training manager responsible for providing consistent quality in programming.

2. All personal trainers receive extensive weight-loss education in their first four weeks of training.

3. We take seriously our position as the top personal training company in Canada. Individual and group training takes place on a daily, weekly, and monthly basis. The focus from day one is on how to be the best.

4. No other company invests as much time and money in staff training as GoodLife.

5. We have five levels of trainers from Motivators to Elite Plus. The level you pick will depend on what satisfies your needs and fits into your budget.

6. Our personal trainers will give you a free half-hour consultation. They will sit down one-on-one and assess your fitness background, needs, and goals. Together you will decide on the best program and time frame for you to accomplish your goals and to look and feel great.

7. With a selection of more than 10 pre-designed programs, we can ensure that you can find the program that is best for you.

8. To keep our trainers leaders in the fitness industry, we pride ourselves in offering extensive training on all aspects of

fitness and wellness. Every personal trainer attends four to six workshops per year. They perform a practical component to stay abreast of the latest fitness research, and complete an exam where they must achieve an 80 percent or higher grade.

9. GoodLife's National Member Services Department constantly researches the latest and most popular trends in education, programming, and coaching skills, helping both staff and members achieve new paths of excellence and growth in their personal and professional life.

10. This same department has excellent international relationships throughout the fitness industry, sharing concepts and techniques with other leaders in this profession.

11. In addition to in-house training, Goodlife's personal trainers have access to a website that provides hundreds of ways to grow and improve a trainer's skill by means of question and answer segments; programming and assessment information; handouts for clients; and hard to find information on specific injuries and chronic problems.

12. To keep our trainers consistent, we publish bimonthly newsletters with articles, research materials, recipes, coaching materials, and testimonials from members and trainers.

13. Many of our trainers attend the GoodLife Fitness and Leadership Conference each year, focused on new industry developments for helping clients.

14. GoodLife continually collects member surveys to ensure that we are always aware of our clients' needs.

15. We have designed a one-of-a-kind preventative Healthy Heart training program to address Canada's number one health concern.

16. We take heart conditioning so seriously that we have installed high-quality blood pressure units in every club so our members can keep track of their heart strength and take measures to keep their hearts young.

17. Feedback as to what members want in personal training is

presented, discussed, and implemented at monthly meetings of our Personal Training Advisory Board.

18. This career is so personally rewarding that it attracts professionals such as teachers, massage therapists, chiropractors, doctors, bankers, and lawyers. The common thread is people who believe in the value of fitness and are committed to helping people feel great and live a better life. Personal trainers at GoodLife care!

And the Big Bonus? Personal training is fun! It's nice to have someone who cares about you, motivates you, and is your "coach." It's great to have someone pat you on the back; it's great to have someone looking out for your fitness and health. Do yourself a favour — try personal training. Even if it requires cutting something else out of your budget, this is absolutely one of the best things you can do for yourself. As I said, I use a personal trainer — I love it and I pay for it. It's one of the best investments I have ever made.

SIX-WEEK FAT LOSS PROGRAM
The results of the Fat Loss Program are truly spectacular!

Women:
lose 9-12 pounds of fat
6-11 inches off in total
2-3 inches off waist, hips, and thighs
add 2-4 pounds of body-shaping muscle to boost metabolism
increase strength 40-100 percent

Men:
lose 13-19 pounds of fat
6-11 inches off in total
2-4 inches off trouble spots — waist and hips
build 3-4 pounds of muscle
50-100 percent increase in strength

Best of all you have a 100 percent money back guarantee, if you do not achieve results from the program.

The Six-Week Fat Loss Program is a signature program of GoodLife Fitness Clubs. It is our most successful program and the one that we're most proud of, which is why we guarantee these remarkable results. This wonderful and exclusive program offers you:

• 18 one-on-one workout sessions, plus pre- and post-fitness assessments.

• One-on-one personal trainers to ensure that you achieve maximum muscular strength on each exercise.

• A nutrition plan that provides daily menus, recipes, and weekly shopping lists. Meal plans are available for all lifestyles: "on the run," vegetarian, etc.

Great results! Less fat! More muscle! What could be better?
Let me tell you a bit about how strength training helps you lose fat and keep it off. Adults lose five to seven pounds of muscle every decade and experience a 10 percent metabolic decrease every decade. Here's what happens when you do strength training in the Fat Loss Program:

• You will add three pounds of lean weight (muscle mass) after six weeks of strength training.

• Three pounds of additional lean weight is associated with a 7 percent increase in your resting metabolic rate.

• You will increase bone mineral density.

• You will reduce your resting blood pressure.

• You will reduce low back pain and ease the pain of osteoarthritis and rheumatoid arthritis.

The Fat Loss Program works. It increases your muscle tissue, which in turn increases your metabolism, which increases the caloric expenditure while at rest and while active (you get a double reducing effect). You get consistency with your workouts —

three times per week. You learn proper and healthy eating habits. Your one-on-one personal trainer provides unparalleled motivation and coaching that allows for a successful completion of each high-intensity workout. The Fat Loss Program is so effective at producing permanent fat loss because it addresses five very important areas.

1. *It manages your dietary calories.*
Dietary calories are the backbone of any successful fat-loss program. The Fat Loss Program includes a six-week eating plan. Men average 1,600 to 1,767 calories per day and women average 1,300 to1,450 calories per day. The proportions of carbohydrates, fats, and proteins are professionally selected to remain constant throughout the daily menus: 50 percent carbohydrates, 30 percent fats, 20 percent proteins. The meal plans are not a fad. They teach you how to eat balanced proper meals so that when you've completed the six-week program, you'll have acquired the knowledge to continue with these great eating habits.

2. *You burn calories.*
The calorie-burning potential of weight-training exercise is second to none. It not only burns calories while you do the exercise, but it also burns calories while you're resting!

3. *It builds muscle mass.*
Traditionally, there have been two ways to lose fat: decrease your dietary calories and increase your exercise to burn calories. The Fat Loss Program promotes the third most successful way: cause your body to use more calories in ways that do not involve exertion.
This third but primary way to burn calories at rest is by building your muscles. By adding one pound of muscle, your body automatically requires an additional 50 calories per day. During the six-week program, the average man adds four pounds of muscle and the average woman adds three-and-a-half pounds. This

extra muscle mass raises your fat-burning metabolism, I believe by 150 to 200 calories a day. That's about a pound every 15 days. It also improves your physical appearance. Most important, building muscle increases your probability of keeping the lost fat off permanently. Weight-training exercises remain the safest, most efficient way to stimulate your muscles to grow larger and stronger. In fact, if you diet without weight training, 80 percent of the weight you lose is muscle, not fat. Weight train and you will lose fat!

4. *You receive proper supervision.*

The personal training and dietary supervision you receive in the Fat Loss Program keeps you on track and motivated. This consistent encouragement and supervision of your program keeps you moving in the direction of your goals and increases your confidence in your ability to lose fat and keep it off.

5. *The program provides maintenance and follow-up.*

Ninety-eight percent of people who only diet to lose significant amounts of fat, without doing strength training, will gain the weight back within the first year. The key to keeping your lost fat off is building muscle. The Fat Loss Program provides the necessary guidelines and follow-up on how to stay at your optimum level for the rest of your life.

HEALTHY HEART PROGRAM

Our Healthy Heart program is the only one of its kind, and I am passionate about sharing the benefits of a healthy heart with you! It is my hope that I can help thousands of Canadians fight heart disease. The goal of this program is to educate you on all the controllable aspects regarding the care of your heart. We take you through the various ways to measure your heart health and how you should exercise to good health. I felt it was important to design a "preventative program," a solution that will help you be proactive now, against heart disease.

The program is designed to educate as many people as possible on the various measures they can take to ensure they have the healthiest heart possible. The program goes through the controllable factors or measures clients can take to help prevent onset of heart disease. Topics covered include controlling stress, nutrition, lifestyle/ habits, cardiovascular training, strength training, and goal setting. Healthy Heart coaches train clients to an excellent level of health in just eight short weeks. We give you a gift of a heart rate monitor and the peace of mind that comes from knowing you are conditioning your heart. Benefits include improved circulation, decreased cholesterol, a stronger heart, and decreased blood pressure.

Afterwards, help is offered to maintain this excellent level of health by having you meet with your coach once a month for up to a year. During this time, reassessments take place to make sure you have maintained your heart strength. The regular checkups will help keep you motivated to work out for years to come!

SUCCESS STORIES CHALLENGE

The Success Stories Challenge is a monthly contest designed to recognize the outstanding achievements our members accomplish through Personal Training, our exclusive Fat Loss Program, our Healthy Heart Program, and our specialty programs. One female and one male winner are chosen monthly to win a $1,000 cash prize! We hope that the results and testimonials submitted will help inspire others to reach for their dreams and achieve their goals. All members are welcome to enter and are encouraged to do so. It doesn't matter whether you're fit or unfit, 16 or 75. It is our hope that this contest, along with the assistance of our Personal Trainers, will inspire you to realize the power and ability within yourself to achieve the goals you desire.

Indoor Tanning — looks good and it's good for you

HAVE YOU EVER NOTICED that people are happier in the sunshine? Have you noticed that people are happier in the summer? Have you also noticed that if people get outside in the winter, whether tobogganing or skiing, they're happier? It's got something to do with both fresh air and sunshine. Real or artificial sunlight assists your body with its production of Vitamin D3 — key for calcium absorption. The most reliable source of Vitamin D is moderate exposure to sunlight and Vitamin D has been associated with a wide variety of health benefits including a reduced rate of death from certain cancers. Studies have shown that tanning reduces stress, blood pressure, serum cholesterol, and resting heart rate.

So if you want to feel good and you want to look good at the same time, do a little tanning — not too much, not too little, just the right balance.

At GoodLife Fitness Clubs we have a 200-page manual on how to offer smart and effective year-round tanning. Our membership in the International Smart Tan Network allows us to attend various events and workshops to gain further education on the benefits of "smart tanning." Together we promote the same simple premise in tanning: moderate tanning for individuals who can develop a tan is the best way to maximize the benefits of sun exposure, while minimizing the risks of either too much or too little exposure.

Evidence shows that sunlight produces metabolic effects in the body that resemble that of physical training. When exposure to ultraviolet light is combined with exercise, your respiratory rate decreases; there is less lactic acid accumulated in the blood; the blood carries oxygen more efficiently; and your heart efficiency increases. Aside from the numerous physiological benefits of tanning, most tanners also experience increased levels of psychological well being. Sunlight and simulated sunlight doses have also shown to be a successful treatment for SAD (seasonal affective disorder), a condition that causes winter depression. Taking time to relax and treat your body to the experience of tanning contributes to improved physical health and general happiness.

With premium, high intensity indoor tanning equipment at nearly every GoodLife Fitness location, you have the convenience of choosing the level of bed you'd prefer to use. You can relax and lie down for up to 20 minutes to get away from daily stress or get in and out in 6-10 minutes for a quick session in our standup beds. Each tanning bed uses a carefully controlled mix of both UVA and UVB ultraviolet light rays to help prevent indoor tanners from burning as easily or as quickly as they could by tanning outdoors. Tanning outdoors does not give the control as indoor tanning does, because the sun emits the entire spectrum of ultraviolet light, including the most intense rays that burn you more quickly. Indoors you have control, since you always know exactly what kind of ultraviolet light you are getting and how long you'll be in the tanning session. You also have the convenience of never having to worry about bad weather or about over-exposure to sunlight. That's why we call indoor tanning "smart tanning."

Here's a layman's description of the entire process: Tanning takes place in the skin's outermost layer, the epidermis. About five percent of the cells in your epidermis are special cells called melanocytes. Melanocytes produce melanin, a brown pigment that is absorbed by all the surrounding skin cells in the epidermis. Once absorbed into a skin cell, melanin actually "enshrouds" the cell's inner material, colouring the cell brown and protecting it from too much ultraviolet light exposure. This process produces a tan — a browning of the skin — that many people throughout the world find cosmetically pleasing. Since tanning is your body's natural defence against sunburn, a cosmetic tan helps to minimize the risk of skin damage.

Tanning at GoodLife gives you the advantage of speed and

convenience. It only takes only a few quick sessions per week to achieve and maintain a golden brown tan. GoodLife also carries a full line of premium indoor tanning lotions that not only help increase the tanning process, but also help to keep the skin healthy and moisturized. Healthy, moisturized skin tans faster and you keep your great glow longer.

You will receive excellent and professional service at the GoodLife Fitness Clubs, as our trained and qualified Customer Service Representatives evaluate your skin type and complete a skin-type analysis when you start to tan. We make recommendations for tanning-session lengths, continually monitor your tan's progress, and advise you on how to properly maintain your tan. Our priority is to get you great smart tanning results.

It makes perfect sense

IT MAKES PERFECT SENSE to take care of yourself. It makes perfect sense to have the very best in fitness training and services. It makes perfect sense to be healthy and fit, to have the Good Life. At GoodLife Fitness Clubs, our excellent and highly qualified staff pride themselves on getting to know your individual needs and on helping you achieve your goals. Together, we're a great team!

> *Remember:*
> *Say to yourself: If it's to be, it's up to me.*
> *Don't let the things you can't do get in the way of the things you can do.*
> *Believe it — Achieve it.*
> *You CAN live the Good Life!*